Preface

The purpose of this pocket reference is to provide you with a handy, easy-to-use manual that is needed to interpret basic dysrhythmias. This reference is intended to accompany the *ECGs Made Easy* textbook. A brief description of most rhythms discussed in the textbook appears in this reference. Each description is accompanied by a summary of the characteristics of the rhythm and a sample rhythm strip. All rhythm strips were recorded in lead II unless otherwise noted. Possible patient signs and symptoms related to the rhythm and treatment options are included in the *ECGs Made Easy* textbook. Every attempt has been made to provide information that is consistent with current literature, including current resuscitation guidelines.

I hope you find this pocket reference of assistance, and I wish you success in your studies.

Best regards,
Barbara Aehlert

Acknowledgments

I would like to thank the manuscript reviewers for their comments and suggestions, which helped to improve the clarity of the information presented in this text, and the following healthcare professionals who provided many of the rhythm strips used in this book: Andrew Baird, CEP; James Bratcher; Joanna Burgan, CEP; Holly Button, CEP; Gretchen Chalmers, CEP; Thomas Cole, CEP; Brent Haines, CEP; Paul Honeywell, CEP; Timothy Klatt, RN; Bill Loughran, RN; Andrea Lowrey, RN; Joe Martinez, CEP; Stephanos Orphanidis, CEP; Jason Payne, CEP; Steve Ruehs, CEP; Patty Seneski, RN; David Stockton, CEP; Jason Stodghill, CEP; Dionne Socie, CEP; Kristina Tellez, CEP; and Fran Wojculewicz, RN.

I would also like to thank the editorial and production teams at Elsevier who continue to provide helpful guidance, humor, and support throughout the development and production of this book and its ancillary materials.

About the Author

Barbara Aehlert, RN, BSPA, is the President of Southwest EMS Education, Inc. She has been a registered nurse for more than 35 years with clinical experience in medical/surgical and critical care nursing and prehospital education. Barbara is an active CPR, First Aid, Paramedic, ACLS, and PALS instructor and takes a special interest in teaching basic dysrhythmia recognition and ACLS to nurses and paramedics.

Pocket Reference for

ECGs MADE EASY

Barbara Aehlert, RN, BSPA
Southwest EMS Education, Inc.

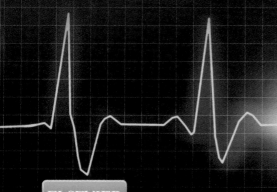

ELSEVIER

Fifth Edition

3251 Riverport Lane
St. Louis, Missouri 63043

POCKET REFERENCE FOR ECGs MADE EASY,
FIFTH EDITION   978-0-323-10108-0

Notices

Knowledge and best practice in this field are constantly changing. As new research and experience broaden our understanding, changes in research methods, professional practices, or medical treatment may become necessary.

Practitioners and researchers must always rely on their own experience and knowledge in evaluating and using any information, methods, compounds, or experiments described herein. In using such information or methods they should be mindful of their own safety and the safety of others, including parties for whom they have a professional responsibility.

With respect to any drug or pharmaceutical products identified, readers are advised to check the most current information provided (i) on procedures featured or (ii) by the manufacturer of each product to be administered, to verify the recommended dose or formula, the method and duration of administration, and contraindications. It is the responsibility of practitioners, relying on their own experience and knowledge of their patients, to make diagnoses, to determine dosages and the best treatment for each individual patient, and to take all appropriate safety precautions.

To the fullest extent of the law, neither the Publisher nor the authors, contributors, or editors, assume any liability for any injury and/or damage to persons or property as a matter of products liability, negligence or otherwise, or from any use or operation of any methods, products, instructions, or ideas contained in the material herein.

978-0-323-10108-0

Executive Content Strategist: Jennifer Janson
Associate Content Development Specialist: Andrea Hunolt
Publishing Services Manager: Julie Eddy
Senior Project Manager: Andrea Campbell
Design Direction: Maggie Reid

Printed in China

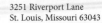

Working together to grow
libraries in developing countries

www.elsevier.com | www.bookaid.org | www.sabre.org

ELSEVIER   BOOK AID International   Sabre Foundation

Last digit is the print number: 9 8 7 6 5 4 3 2 1

Contents

Contents

Anatomy and Physiology

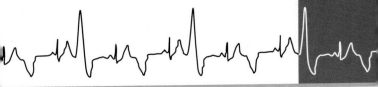

LOCATION AND SURFACES OF THE HEART

The heart is a hollow muscular organ that lies in the space between the lungs (i.e., the mediastinum) in the middle of the chest. It sits behind the sternum and just above the diaphragm (Figure 1-1). Approximately two thirds of the heart lie to the left of the midline of the sternum. The remaining third lies to the right of the sternum.

The base, or posterior surface, of the heart is formed by the left atrium, a small portion of the right atrium, and proximal portions of the superior and inferior venae cavae and the pulmonary veins. The front (anterior) surface of the heart lies behind the sternum and costal cartilages. It is formed by portions of the right atrium and the left and right ventricles (Figure 1-2). The heart's apex, or lower portion, is formed by the tip of the left ventricle. The apex lies just above the diaphragm at approximately the level of the fifth intercostal space, in the midclavicular line.

STRUCTURE OF THE HEART

Layers of the Heart Wall

The walls of the heart are made up of three tissue layers: the endocardium, myocardium, and epicardium. The heart's innermost layer, the endocardium, is made up of a thin, smooth layer of epithelium and connective tissue and lines the heart's inner chambers, valves, chordae tendineae (tendinous cords), and papillary muscles. The endocardium is continuous with the

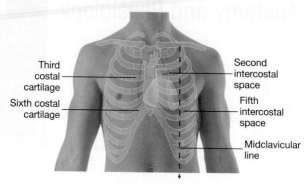

Figure 1-1 Anterior view of the chest wall of a man showing skeletal structures and the surface projection of the heart.

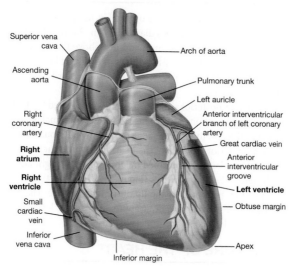

Figure 1-2 The anterior surface of the heart.

innermost layer of the arteries, veins, and capillaries of the body, thereby creating a continuous, closed circulatory system. The myocardium (middle layer) is a thick, muscular layer that consists of cardiac muscle fibers (cells) responsible for the pumping action of the heart. The heart's outermost layer is called the *epicardium*. The epicardium contains blood capillaries, lymph capillaries, nerve fibers, and fat.

Heart Chambers

The heart has four chambers (Figure 1-3). The two upper chambers are the right and left atria. The purpose of the atria is to receive blood. The right atrium receives blood low in oxygen from the superior vena cava (which carries blood from the head and upper extremities), the inferior vena cava (which carries blood from the lower body), and the coronary sinus, which is the largest vein that drains the heart. The left atrium receives freshly oxygenated blood from the lungs via the right and left pulmonary veins.

The heart's two lower chambers are the right and left ventricles. Their purpose is to pump blood. The right ventricle pumps blood to the lungs. The left ventricle pumps blood out to the body.

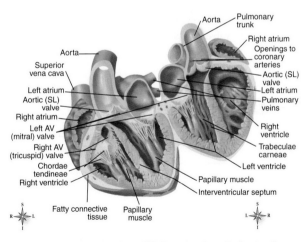

Figure 1-3 Interior of the heart. This illustration shows the heart as it would appear if it were cut along a frontal plane and opened like a book. The front portion of the heart lies to the reader's right; the back portion of the heart lies to the reader's left. (Note each portion has a separate anatomical rosette to facilitate orientation.) The four chambers of the heart—two atria and two ventricles—are easily seen. AV, atrioventricular; SL, semilunar.

Heart Valves

There are four one-way valves in the heart: two sets of atrio-ventricular (AV) valves and two sets of semilunar (SL) valves (Table 1-1). The valves open and close in a specific sequence and assist in producing the pressure gradient needed between the chambers to ensure a smooth flow of blood through the heart and prevent the backflow of blood.

AV valves separate the atria from the ventricles. The tricuspid valve is the AV valve that lies between the right atrium and right ventricle. It consists of three separate cusps or flaps. It is larger in diameter and thinner than the mitral valve. The mitral (or bicuspid) valve has only two cusps. It lies between the left atrium and left ventricle.

The pulmonic and aortic valves are SL valves. The SL valves prevent backflow of blood from the aorta and pulmonary arteries into the ventricles. The SL valves have three cusps shaped like half-moons. The openings of the SL valves are smaller than the openings of the AV valves and the flaps of the SL valves are smaller and thicker than the AV valves. Unlike the AV valves, the SL valves are not attached to chordae tendineae.

Table **1-1**	Heart Valves		
Valve Type	Name	Right Heart vs. Left Heart	Location
Atrioventricular	Tricuspid	Right	Separates right atrium and right ventricle
	Mitral (Bicuspid)	Left	Separates left atrium and left ventricle
Semilunar	Pulmonic	Right	Between right ventricle and pulmonary artery
	Aortic	Left	Between left ventricle and aorta

THE HEART'S BLOOD SUPPLY

The coronary circulation consists of coronary arteries and veins. The main coronary arteries lie on the outer (epicardial) surface of the heart. The three major coronary arteries include the left anterior descending (LAD) artery, circumflex (CX) artery, and the right coronary artery (RCA) (Figure 1-4, Table 1-2). A person is said to have coronary artery disease (CAD) if there is more than 50% diameter narrowing (i.e., stenosis) in one or more of these vessels.

The coronary (cardiac) veins travel alongside the arteries. The coronary sinus is the largest vein that drains the heart. It lies in the groove that separates the atria from the ventricles. Blood that has passed through the myocardial capillaries is drained by branches of the cardiac veins that join the coronary sinus.

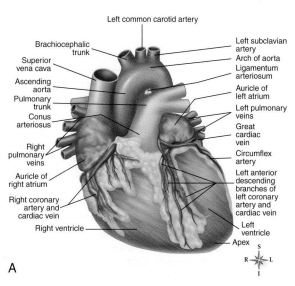

Figure 1-4 The heart and great vessels. **A,** Anterior view of the heart and great vessels.

Continued

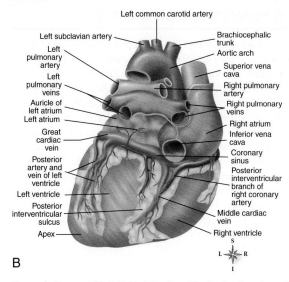

Left common carotid artery

Left subclavian artery

Left pulmonary artery

Left pulmonary veins

Auricle of left atrium

Left atrium

Great cardiac vein

Posterior artery and vein of left ventricle

Left ventricle

Posterior interventricular sulcus

Apex

Brachiocephalic trunk

Aortic arch

Superior vena cava

Right pulmonary artery

Right pulmonary veins

Right atrium

Inferior vena cava

Coronary sinus

Posterior interventricular branch of right coronary artery

Middle cardiac vein

Right ventricle

B

Figure 1-4, cont'd   B, Posterior view of the heart and great vessels.

ACUTE CORONARY SYNDROMES

Acute coronary syndrome (ACS) is a term used to refer to distinct conditions caused by a similar sequence of pathologic events and that involve a temporary or permanent blockage of a coronary artery. This sequence of events results in conditions that range from myocardial ischemia or injury to death (i.e., necrosis) of the heart muscle. The usual cause of an ACS is the rupture of an atherosclerotic plaque. *Arteriosclerosis* is a chronic disease of the arterial system characterized by abnormal thickening and hardening of the vessel walls. *Atherosclerosis* is a form of arteriosclerosis in which the thickening and hardening of the vessel walls are caused by a buildup of fat-like deposits (e.g., plaque) in the inner lining of large and middle-sized muscular arteries. As the fatty deposits build up, the opening of the artery slowly narrows and blood flow to the muscle decreases (Figure 1-5). Complete blockage of a coronary artery may cause a heart attack, also called a *myocardial infarction* (MI).

Table 1-2	Coronary Arteries	
Coronary Artery	Portion of Myocardium Supplied	Portion of Conduction System Supplied
Right	• Right atrium • Right ventricle • Inferior surface of left ventricle (about 85%*) • Posterior surface of left ventricle (85%*)	• Sinoatrial (SA) node (in about 60%*) • Atrioventricular (AV) bundle (85% to 90%*)
Left anterior descending	• Anterior surface of left ventricle • Part of lateral surface of left ventricle • Anterior two thirds of interventricular septum	• Most of right bundle branch • Anterior-superior fascicle of left bundle branch • Part of posterior-inferior fascicle of left bundle branch
Circumflex	• Left atrium • Part of lateral surface of left ventricle • Inferior surface of left ventricle (about 15%*) • Posterior surface of left ventricle (15%*)	• SA node (about 40%*) • AV bundle (10% to 15%*)

*Of population.

Angina pectoris is chest discomfort or other related symptoms of sudden onset that may occur because the increased oxygen demand of the heart temporarily exceeds the blood supply. Angina is not a disease. Rather, it is a symptom of myocardial ischemia. Angina most often occurs in patients with CAD that involves at least one coronary artery. However, it can be present in patients with normal coronary arteries. Angina also occurs in persons with uncontrolled high blood pressure or valvular heart disease. Chest discomfort associated with myocardial ischemia usually begins in the central or left chest and then radiates to the arm (especially the little finger [ulnar] side of the left arm), the wrist, the jaw, the epigastrium, the left shoulder, or between the shoulder blades.

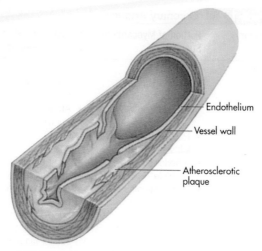

Endothelium

Vessel wall

Atherosclerotic plaque

Figure 1-5 Partial blockage of an artery in atherosclerosis. Atherosclerotic plaque develops from the deposition of fats and other substances in the wall of the artery.

Ischemia prolonged for more than just a few minutes results in myocardial injury. *Myocardial injury* refers to myocardial tissue that has been cut off from or has experienced a severe reduction in its blood and oxygen supply. Injured myocardial cells are still alive but will die (i.e., *infarct*) if the ischemia is not quickly corrected. An MI occurs when blood flow to the heart muscle stops or is suddenly decreased long enough to cause cell death. If the blocked coronary vessel can be quickly opened to restore blood flow and oxygen to the injured area, no tissue death occurs. Methods to restore blood flow may include giving clot-busting drugs (fibrinolytics), performing coronary angioplasty, or performing a coronary artery bypass graft (CABG), among others.

THE HEART AS A PUMP

The right and left sides of the heart are separated by an internal wall of connective tissue called a *septum*. The *interatrial septum* separates the right and left atria. The *interventricular septum* separates the right and left ventricles. The septa separate the heart into two functional pumps. The right atrium and right ventricle make up one pump. The left atrium and left ventricle make up the other (Figure 1-6).

The right side of the heart is a low-pressure system whose job is to pump unoxygenated blood from the body to and through the lungs to the left side of the heart. This is called the *pulmonary circulation*. The job of the left heart is to receive oxygenated blood from the lungs and pump it out to the rest of the body. This is called the *systemic circulation*. Blood is carried from the heart to the organs of the body through arteries, arterioles, and capillaries. Blood is returned to the right heart through venules and veins.

Cardiac Cycle

The cardiac cycle refers to a repetitive pumping process that includes all of the events associated with blood flow through the heart. The cycle has two phases for each heart chamber: systole and diastole. Systole is the period during which the chamber is contracting and blood is being ejected. *Systole* includes contraction of both atrial and ventricular muscle. *Diastole* is the period of relaxation during which the chambers are allowed to fill. The

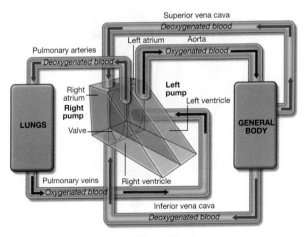

Figure 1-6   The heart has two pumps.

myocardium receives its fresh supply of oxygenated blood from the coronary arteries during ventricular diastole.

During the cardiac cycle, the pressure within each chamber of the heart rises in systole and falls in diastole. The heart's valves ensure that blood flows in the proper direction. Blood flows from one heart chamber to another if the pressure in the chamber is more than the pressure in the next. These pressure relationships depend on the careful timing of contractions. The heart's conduction system provides the necessary timing of events between atrial and ventricular systole.

The right atrium receives blood low in oxygen and high in carbon dioxide from the superior and inferior vena cavae and the coronary sinus (Figure 1-7). Blood flows from the right atrium through the tricuspid valve into the right ventricle.

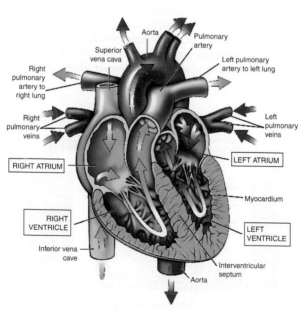

Figure 1-7 Blood flow through the heart.

When the right ventricle contracts, the tricuspid valve closes. The right ventricle expels the blood through the pulmonic valve into the pulmonary trunk. The pulmonary trunk divides into a right and left pulmonary artery, each of which carries blood to one lung (pulmonary circuit). Blood flows through the pulmonary arteries to the lungs (where oxygen and carbon dioxide are exchanged in the pulmonary capillaries) and then to the pulmonary veins. The left atrium receives oxygenated blood from the lungs via the four pulmonary veins (two from the right lung and two from the left lung). Blood flows from the left atrium through the mitral (bicuspid) valve into the left ventricle. When the left ventricle contracts, the mitral valve closes. Blood leaves the left ventricle through the aortic valve to the aorta and its branches and is distributed throughout the body (systemic circuit). Blood from the tissues of the head, neck, and upper extremities is emptied into the superior vena cava. Blood from the lower body is emptied into the inferior vena cava. The superior and inferior vena cavae carry their blood into the right atrium.

The mechanical activity of the heart is reflected by the pulse and blood pressure. *Blood pressure* is the force exerted by the circulating blood volume on the walls of the arteries. The volume of blood in the arteries is directly related to arterial blood pressure. Blood pressure is equal to cardiac output × peripheral resistance. *Peripheral resistance* is the resistance to the flow of blood determined by blood vessel diameter and the tone of the vascular musculature. Blood pressure is affected by conditions or medications that affect peripheral resistance or cardiac output.

Cardiac output is the amount of blood pumped into the aorta each minute by the heart. It is defined as the *stroke volume*, which is the amount of blood ejected from a ventricle with each heartbeat, multiplied by the heart rate. In a healthy average adult, the cardiac output at rest is about 5 L/min. The percentage of blood pumped out of a ventricle with each contraction is called the *ejection fraction*. Ejection fraction is used as a measure of ventricular function. A normal ejection fraction is between 50% and 65%. Signs and symptoms of decreased cardiac output are shown in Box 1-1.

| Box **1-1** | Signs and Symptoms of Decreased Cardiac Output |

- Acute changes in blood pressure
- Acute changes in mental status
- Cold, clammy skin
- Color changes in the skin and mucous membranes
- Crackles (rales)
- Dyspnea
- Dysrhythmias
- Fatigue
- Orthopnea
- Restlessness

Basic Electrophysiology

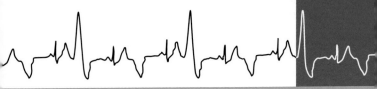

CARDIAC CELLS

Types of Cardiac Cells

In general, cardiac cells have either a mechanical (i.e., contractile) or an electrical (i.e., pacemaker) function. *Myocardial cells* are also called *working cells* or *mechanical cells*, and they contain contractile filaments. When these cells are electrically stimulated, these filaments slide together and cause the myocardial cell to contract. These myocardial cells form the thin muscular layer of the atrial walls and the thicker muscular layer of the ventricular walls (i.e., the myocardium). These cells do not normally generate electrical impulses, and they rely on pacemaker cells for this function.

Pacemaker cells are specialized cells of the electrical conduction system. Pacemaker cells also may be referred to as *conducting cells* or *automatic cells*. They are responsible for the spontaneous generation and conduction of electrical impulses.

Properties of Cardiac Cells

The ability of cardiac pacemaker cells to create an electrical impulse without being stimulated from another source is called *automaticity*. The heart's normal pacemaker is the sinoatrial (SA) node because it is capable of self-excitation at a rate quicker than that of other pacemaker sites in the heart. *Excitability* (i.e., irritability) is the ability of cardiac muscle cells to respond to an external stimulus, such as that from a chemical, mechanical, or electrical source. *Conductivity* is the ability of a cardiac cell to receive an electrical impulse and conduct it to an

13

adjoining cardiac cell. All cardiac cells possess this characteristic. *Contractility* (i.e., inotropy) is the ability of myocardial cells to shorten, thereby causing cardiac muscle contraction in response to an electrical stimulus. The heart normally contracts in response to an impulse that begins in the SA node.

CARDIAC ACTION POTENTIAL

Human body fluids contain *electrolytes*, which are elements or compounds that break into charged particles (*ions*) when melted or dissolved in water or another solvent. Differences in the composition of ions between the intracellular and extracellular fluid compartments are important for normal body function, including the activity of the heart. The main electrolytes that affect the function of the heart are sodium ($Na+$), potassium ($K+$), calcium ($Ca++$), and chloride ($Cl-$).

Electrolytes are quickly moved from one side of the cell membrane to the other by means of pumps. These pumps require energy in the form of adenosine triphosphate (ATP) when movement occurs against a concentration gradient. The energy expended by the cells to move electrolytes across the cell membrane creates a flow of current. This flow of current is expressed in volts. Voltage appears on an electrocardiogram (ECG) as spikes or waveforms

The *action potential* of a cardiac cell reflects the rapid sequence of voltage changes that occur across the cell membrane during the electrical cardiac cycle. The configuration of the action potential varies depending on the location, size, and function of the cardiac cell.

There are two main types of action potentials in the heart (Figure 2-1). The first type, the fast response action potential, occurs in normal atrial and ventricular myocardial cells and in the Purkinje fibers, which are specialized conducting fibers found in both ventricles that conduct an electrical impulse through the heart. The second type of cardiac action potential, the slow response action potential, occurs in the heart's normal pacemaker (i.e., the SA node) and in the atrioventricular (AV) node, which is the specialized conducting tissue that carries an electrical impulse from the atria to the ventricles.

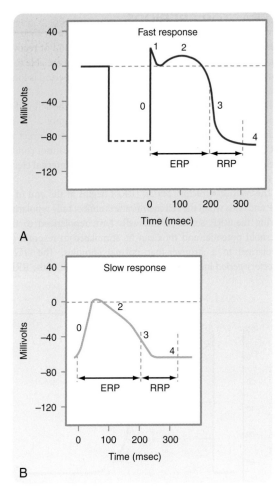

Figure 2-1 Action potentials of fast-response **(A)** and slow-response **(B)** cardiac fibers. The phases of the action potentials are labeled. The effective refractory period (ERP) and the relative refractory period (RRP) are labeled.

REFRACTORY PERIODS

Refractoriness is a term used to describe the period of recovery that cells need after being discharged before they are able to respond to a stimulus. In the heart, the refractory period is longer than the contraction itself.

During the *absolute refractory period* (ARP), the cell will not respond to further stimulation within itself (Figure 2-2). This means that the myocardial working cells cannot contract and that the cells of the electrical conduction system cannot conduct an electrical impulse, no matter how strong the internal electrical stimulus.

The *relative refractory period* (RRP) begins at the end of the ARP and ends when the cell membrane is almost fully repolarized. During the RRP, some cardiac cells have repolarized to their threshold potential and thus can be stimulated to respond (i.e., depolarize) to a stronger-than-normal stimulus. The *effective refractory period* includes the ARP and the first half of the RRP.

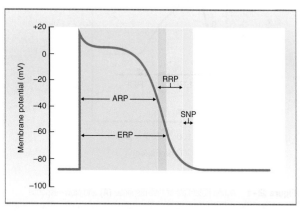

Figure 2-2   Refractory periods of the ventricular action potential. The effective refractory period (ERP) includes the absolute refractory period (ARP) and the first half of the relative refractory period (RRP). The RRP begins when the ARP ends and includes the last portion of the ERP. The supranormal period (SNP) begins when the RRP ends.

After the RRP is a *supranormal* period. A weaker-than-normal stimulus can cause cardiac cells to depolarize during this period. Because the cell is more excitable than normal, dysrhythmias can develop during this period.

CONDUCTION SYSTEM

Figure 2-3 shows the heart's conduction system. A summary of the conduction system is shown in Table 2-1.

Causes of Dysrhythmias

Dysrhythmias result from disorders of impulse formation, disorders of impulse conduction, or both.

Disorders of Impulse Formation
Enhanced Automaticity

Enhanced automaticity is an abnormal condition in which one of the following occurs: (1) Cardiac cells that are not

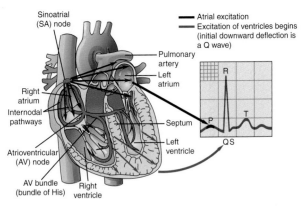

Figure 2-3   Schematic drawing of the conducting system of the heart. An impulse normally is generated in the sinoatrial node and travels through the atria to the AV node, down the bundle of His and Purkinje fibers, and to the ventricular myocardium. Recording of the depolarizing and repolarizing currents in the heart with electrodes on the surface of the body produces characteristic waveforms.

Table 2-1	Summary of the Conduction System			
Structure	Location	Function	Intrinsic Pacemaker (beats/min)	Time Lapse from SA Node (seconds)
Sinoatrial (SA) node	Right atrial wall just inferior to opening of superior vena cava	Primary pacemaker; initiates impulse that is normally conducted throughout the left and right atria	60 to 100	0
Atrioventricular (AV) node	Floor of the right atrium immediately behind the tricuspid valve and near the opening of the coronary sinus	Receives impulse from SA node and delays relay of the impulse to the bundle of His, allowing time for the atria to empty their contents into the ventricles before the onset of ventricular contraction		0.03
Bundle of His (AV bundle)	Superior portion of interventricular septum	Receives impulse from AV node and relays it to right and left bundle branches	40 to 60	0.04
Right and left bundle branches	Interventricular septum	Receives impulse from bundle of His and relays it to Purkinje fibers		0.17
Purkinje fibers	Ventricular myocardium	Receives impulse from bundle branches and relays it to ventricular myocardium	20 to 40	0.20 to 0.22

normally associated with a pacemaker function begin to depolarize spontaneously or (2) a pacemaker site other than the SA node increases its firing rate beyond that which is considered normal.

Triggered Activity

Triggered activity results from abnormal electrical impulses that sometimes occur during repolarization, when cells are normally quiet. These abnormal electrical impulses are called *afterdepolarizations*. Triggered activity requires a stimulus to begin depolarization. It occurs when pacemaker cells from a site other than the SA node and myocardial working cells depolarize more than once after being stimulated by a single impulse.

Disorders of Impulse Conduction
Conduction Blocks

Blocks of impulse conduction may be partial or complete. They may occur because of trauma, drug toxicity, electrolyte disturbances, myocardial ischemia, or infarction. A partial conduction block may be slowed or intermittent. In slowed conduction, all impulses are conducted but it takes longer than normal to do so. When an intermittent block occurs, some (but not all) impulses are conducted. When a complete block exists, no impulses are conducted through the affected area. Examples of rhythms associated with disturbances in conduction include AV blocks.

Reentry

An impulse normally spreads through the heart only once after it is initiated by pacemaker cells. *Reentry* is the spread of an impulse through tissue already stimulated by that same impulse. An electrical impulse is delayed, blocked, or both, in one or more areas of the conduction system while the impulse is conducted normally through the rest of the conduction system (Figure 2-4). This results in the delayed electrical impulse entering cardiac cells that have just been depolarized by the normally conducted impulse. If the area the delayed impulse stimulates is relatively refractory, the impulse can cause depolarization of those cells, producing a single premature beat or repetitive electrical impulses. This can result in short periods of an abnormally fast heart rate.

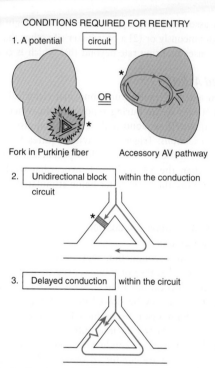

CONDITIONS REQUIRED FOR REENTRY

1. A potential | circuit |

OR

Fork in Purkinje fiber   Accessory AV pathway

2. | Unidirectional block | within the conduction
circuit

3. | Delayed conduction | within the circuit

Figure 2-4   Reentry requires (1) a potential conduction circuit or circular conduction pathway, (2) a block within part of the circuit, and (3) delayed conduction with the remainder of the circuit.

THE ELECTROCARDIOGRAM

Electrocardiogram (ECG) monitoring may be used for the following purposes:
- To monitor a patient's heart rate
- To evaluate the effects of disease or injury on heart function
- To evaluate pacemaker function
- To evaluate the response to medications (e.g., antiarrhythmics)
- To obtain a baseline recording before, during, and after a medical procedure

- To evaluate for signs of myocardial ischemia, injury, and infarction

The ECG *can* provide information about the following:

- The orientation of the heart in the chest
- Conduction disturbances
- Electrical effects of medications and electrolytes
- The mass of cardiac muscle
- The presence of ischemic damage

The ECG does *not* provide information about the mechanical (contractile) condition of the myocardium. To evaluate the effectiveness of the heart's mechanical activity, the patient's pulse and blood pressure are assessed.

Electrodes

Electrode refers to an adhesive pad, containing a conductive substance in the center, that is applied to the patient's skin. The conductive media of the electrode conducts skin surface voltage changes through wires to a cardiac monitor (electrocardiograph). Electrodes are applied at specific locations on the patient's chest wall and extremities to view the heart's electrical activity from different angles and planes. One end of a monitoring cable, which is also called a *lead wire*, is attached to the electrode and the other end to an ECG machine. The cable conducts current back to the cardiac monitor.

Leads

A *lead* is a record (i.e., tracing) of electrical activity between two electrodes. Each lead records the *average* current flow at a specific time in a portion of the heart. Leads allow viewing the heart's electrical activity in two different planes: frontal (coronal) and horizontal (transverse). A 12-lead ECG provides views of the heart in both the frontal and horizontal planes and views the surfaces of the left ventricle from 12 different angles (Figure 2-5). From this, ischemia, injury, and infarction affecting any area of the heart can be identified.

A summary of the standard limb leads can be found in Figure 2-6 and Table 2-2, a summary of the augmented leads appears in Figure 2-7 and Table 2-3, and a summary of the chest leads can be found in Figure 2-8 and Table 2-4.

A   FRONTAL PLANE LEADS

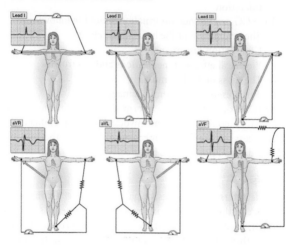

B   HORIZONTAL PLANE—CHEST LEADS

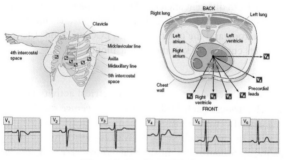

Figure 2-5   The ECG leads.

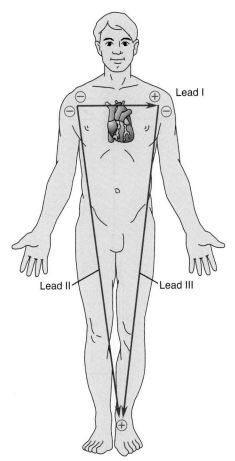

Figure 2-6 Positions of standard limb leads I, II, and III.

Table 2-2	Summary of Standard Limb Leads		
Lead	Positive Electrode	Negative Electrode	Heart Surface Viewed
I	Left arm	Right arm	Lateral
II	Left leg	Right arm	Inferior
III	Left leg	Left arm	Inferior

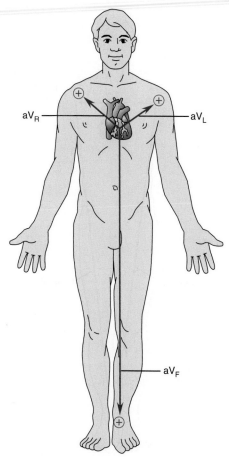

Figure 2-7   Augmented leads aVR, aVL, and aVF.

Table **2-3**	Summary of Augmented Leads	
Lead	Positive Electrode	Heart Surface Viewed
aVR	Right arm	None
aVL	Left arm	Lateral
aVF	Left leg	Inferior

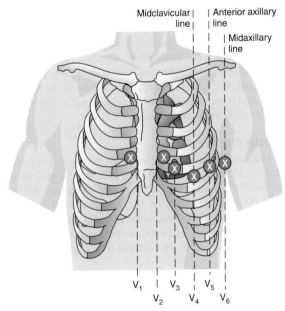

Figure 2-8 Chest (precordial) leads V_1 through V_6.

Table **2-4**	Summary of Chest Leads	
Lead	**Positive Electrode Position**	**Heart Surface Viewed**
V_1	Right side of sternum, fourth intercostal space	Septum
V_2	Left side of sternum, fourth intercostal space	Septum
V_3	Midway between V_2 and V_4	Anterior
V_4	Left midclavicular line, fifth intercostal space	Anterior
V_5	Left anterior axillary line; same level as V_4	Lateral
V_6	Left midaxillary line; same level as V_4	Lateral

Right Chest Leads

Other chest leads that are not part of a standard 12-lead ECG may be used to view specific surfaces of the heart. When a right ventricular myocardial infarction is suspected, right chest leads are used. Placement of right chest leads is identical to placement of the standard chest leads except that it is done on the right side of the chest (Figure 2-9). If time does not permit obtaining all of the right chest leads, the lead of choice is V_4R.

Posterior Chest Leads

On a standard 12-lead ECG, no leads look directly at the posterior surface of the heart. Additional chest leads may be used for this purpose. These leads are placed further left and toward the back. All of the leads are placed on the same horizontal line as V_4 through V_6. Lead V_7 is placed at the posterior axillary line. Lead V_8 is placed at the angle of the scapula (posterior scapular line) and lead V_9 is placed over the left border of spine (Figure 2-10).

Electrocardiography Paper

Remember that the ECG is a graphical representation of the heart's electrical activity. When you place electrodes on the patient's body and connect them to an ECG, the machine records the voltage

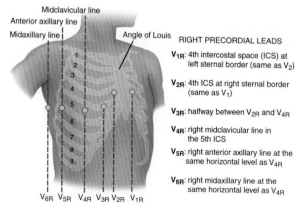

RIGHT PRECORDIAL LEADS

V_{1R}: 4th intercostal space (ICS) at left sternal border (same as V_2)

V_{2R}: 4th ICS at right sternal border (same as V_1)

V_{3R}: halfway between V_{2R} and V_{4R}

V_{4R}: right midclavicular line in the 5th ICS

V_{5R}: right anterior axillary line at the same horizontal level as V_{4R}

V_{6R}: right midaxillary line at the same horizontal level as V_{4R}

Figure 2-9 Electrode locations for recording a right chest ECG. Right chest leads are not of a standard 12-lead ECG but are used when a right ventricular infarction is suspected.

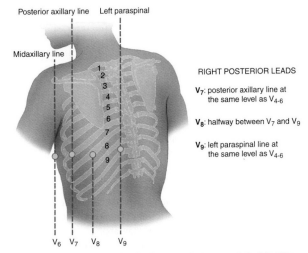

Posterior axillary line   Left paraspinal

Midaxillary line

1
2
3
4
5
6
7
8
9

RIGHT POSTERIOR LEADS

V_7: posterior axillary line at the same level as V_{4-6}

V_8: halfway between V_7 and V_9

V_9: left paraspinal line at the same level as V_{4-6}

V_6 V_7 V_8 V_9

Figure 2-10   Posterior chest leads are used when a posterior infarction is suspected. First obtain and print a standard 12-lead ECG. Then locate the landmarks for the posterior leads: posterior axillary line, midscapular line, and left border of the spine. Leads V_7, V_8, and V_9 are on the same horizontal line as leads V_4, V_5, and V_6 on the front of the chest.

(i.e., the potential difference) between the electrodes. The needle (or pen) of the ECG moves a specific distance depending on the voltage measured. This recording is made on ECG paper.

ECG paper is graph paper made up of small and large boxes measured in millimeters. The smallest boxes are 1-mm wide and 1-mm high (Figure 2-11). The horizontal axis of the paper corresponds with *time*. Time is used to measure the interval between or duration of specific cardiac events, which is stated in seconds.

ECG paper normally records at a constant speed of 25 mm/sec. Thus, each horizontal unit (i.e., each 1-mm box) represents 0.04 second (25 mm/sec × 0.04 second = 1 mm). The lines after every five small boxes on the paper are heavier. The heavier lines indicate one large box. Because each large box is the width of five small boxes, a large box represents 0.20 second. Five large boxes, each consisting of five small boxes, represent 1 second; fifteen large boxes equal an interval of 3 seconds; and thirty large boxes represent 6 seconds.

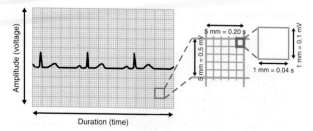

Figure 2-11   Electrocardiograph strip showing the markings for measuring amplitude and duration of waveforms, using a standard recording speed of 25 mm/sec.

The vertical axis of the graph paper represents the voltage or amplitude of the ECG waveforms or deflections. Voltage is measured in millivolts (mV). Voltage may appear as a positive or negative value, because voltage is a force with direction as well as amplitude. Amplitude is measured in millimeters (mm). The ECG machine's sensitivity must be calibrated so that a 1-mV electrical signal will produce a deflection that measures exactly 10-mm tall. When properly calibrated, a small box is 1 mm high (i.e., 0.1 mV), and a large box, which is equal to five small boxes, is 5 mm high (i.e., 0.5 mV). Clinically, the height of a waveform is usually stated in millimeters rather than in millivolts.

WAVEFORMS

A *waveform* (i.e., a deflection) is movement away from the baseline in a positive (i.e., upward) or negative (i.e., downward) direction. Each waveform seen on an ECG is related to a specific electrical event in the heart. Waveforms are named alphabetically, beginning with P, QRS, T, and U. When electrical activity is not detected, a straight line is recorded. This line is called the *baseline* or *isoelectric line*.

P Wave

Activation of the SA node occurs before the onset of the P wave. This event is not recorded on the ECG. However, the spread of that impulse throughout the atria (atrial depolarization) is observed. The first waveform in the cardiac cycle is the P wave

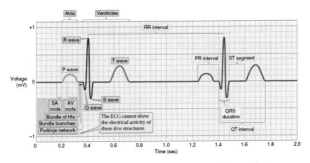

Figure 2-12 Components of the ECG recording. AV, Atrioventricular; SA, sinoatrial.

(Figure 2-12). The beginning of the P wave is recognized as the first abrupt or gradual movement away from the baseline; its end is the point at which the waveform returns to the baseline. The first half of the P wave is recorded when the electrical impulse that originated in the SA node stimulates the right atrium and reaches the AV node. The downslope of the P wave reflects stimulation of the left atrium; thus the P wave represents atrial depolarization and the spread of the electrical impulse throughout the right and left atria. A P wave normally precedes each QRS complex.

QRS Complex

A *complex* consists of several waveforms. The QRS complex consists of the Q wave, R wave, and S wave and represents the spread of the electrical impulse through the ventricles (i.e., ventricular depolarization) and the sum of all ventricular muscle cell depolarizations. Ventricular depolarization normally triggers contraction of ventricular tissue. Thus, shortly after the QRS complex begins, the ventricles contract.

The QRS duration is a measurement of the time required for ventricular depolarization. The width of a QRS complex is most accurately determined when it is viewed and measured in more than one lead. The measurement should be taken from the QRS complex with the longest duration and clearest onset and end. The beginning of the QRS complex is measured from the point where the first wave of the complex begins to deviate from the baseline. The point at which the last wave of the complex begins to level out or distinctly change direction at, above, or below the baseline marks the end of the QRS complex. In adults, the normal duration of the QRS complex is 0.11 second or less. If an electrical impulse does not follow the normal ventricular conduction pathway, it will take longer to depolarize the myocardium. This delay in conduction through the ventricle produces a wider QRS complex.

T Wave

Ventricular repolarization is represented on the ECG by the T wave. The ARP is still present during the beginning of the T wave. At the peak of the T wave, the RRP has begun. It is during the RRP that a stronger-than-normal stimulus may produce ventricular dysrhythmias.

The normal T wave is slightly asymmetric: the peak of the waveform is closer to its end than to the beginning, and the first half has a more gradual slope than the second half. The beginning of the T wave is identified as the point where the slope of the ST segment appears to become abruptly or gradually steeper. The T wave ends when it returns to the baseline. The direction of the T wave is normally the same as the QRS complex that precedes it.

U Wave

A U wave is a small waveform that, when seen, follows the T wave. The U wave represents repolarization of the Purkinje fibers in the papillary muscle of the ventricular myocardium. Normal U waves are small, round, and symmetric. U waves are most easily seen when the heart rate is slow, and they are difficult to identify when the rate exceeds 95 beats/min. U waves usually appear in the same direction as the T waves that precede them.

SEGMENTS

A segment is a line between waveforms. It is named by the waveform that precedes or follows it.

PR Segment

The PR segment is part of the PR interval—specifically, the horizontal line between the end of the P wave and the beginning of the QRS complex. The PR segment is normally isoelectric and represents the spread of the electrical impulse from the AV node, through the AV bundle, right and left bundle branches, and the Purkinje fibers.

TP Segment

The TP segment is the portion of the ECG tracing between the end of the T wave and the beginning of the following P wave during which there is no electrical activity (Figure 2-13). When the heart rate is within normal limits, the TP segment is usually isoelectric and used as the reference point from which to estimate the position of the isoelectric line and determine ST-segment displacement.

ST Segment

The portion of the ECG tracing between the QRS complex and the T wave is the ST segment. The term *ST segment* is used

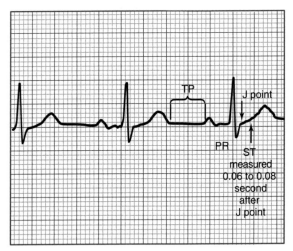

Figure 2-13 The TP segment is used as the reference point for the isoelectric line if the heart rate is slow enough for the TP interval to be clearly seen.

regardless of whether the final wave of the QRS complex is an R or an S wave. The ST segment represents the early part of repolarization of the right and left ventricles. The normal ST segment begins at the isoelectric line, extends from the end of the S wave, and curves gradually upward to the beginning of the T wave. In the limb leads, the normal ST segment is isoelectric (flat) but may normally be slightly elevated or depressed.

The point where the QRS complex and the ST segment meet is called the *ST junction* or the *J point*. The ST segment is considered elevated if the segment is deviated above the baseline, it is considered depressed if the segment deviates below it. When looking for ST-segment elevation or depression, first locate the J point. Next use the TP segment to estimate the position of the isoelectric line. Then compare the level of the ST segment with the isoelectric line. Deviation is measured as the number of millimeters of vertical ST-segment displacement from the isoelectric line or from the patient's baseline at a point 0.06 or 0.08 second after the J point.

INTERVALS

PR Interval

An *interval* is made up of a waveform and a segment. The P wave plus the PR segment equals the PR interval (PRI). Remember that the P wave reflects depolarization of the right and left atria. The PR segment represents the spread of the impulse through the AV node, AV bundle, right and left bundle branches, and the Purkinje fibers. The PRI does not reflect the duration of conduction from the SA node to the right atrium.

The PRI is measured from the point where the P wave leaves the baseline to the beginning of the QRS complex. The term *PQ interval* is preferred by some, because it is the period that is actually measured unless a Q wave is absent. The PRI changes with heart rate but normally measures 0.12 to 0.20 second in adults. As the heart rate increases, the duration of the PRI shortens. A PRI is considered *short* if it is less than 0.12 second and *long* if it is more than 0.20 second.

QT Interval

The QT interval is the period from the beginning of the QRS complex to the end of the T wave. It represents total ventricular activity; this is the time from ventricular depolarization (i.e., activation) to repolarization (i.e., recovery). When measuring the QT interval, first select a lead with the most clearly defined T-wave end. To ensure meaningful comparisons of later tracings, use the same lead for subsequent measurements. In the absence of a Q wave, the QT interval is measured from the beginning of the R wave to the end of the T wave. The term *QT interval* is used regardless of whether the QRS complex begins with a Q wave or an R wave.

The duration of the QT interval varies in accordance with age, gender, and heart rate. As the heart rate increases, the QT interval shortens (i.e., decreases). As the heart rate decreases, the QT interval lengthens (i.e., increases). To quickly estimate the QT interval, first measure the interval between two consecutive R waves (R-R interval). If the measured QT interval is less than half the R-R interval of that QRS complex and the R wave of the following complex, it is probably normal (provided the patient's heart rate is 95 beats/min or less).

R-R and P-P Intervals

The R-R (R wave-to-R wave) and P-P (P wave-to-P wave) intervals are used to determine the rate and rhythmicity (regularity) of a cardiac rhythm. To evaluate the rhythmicity of the ventricular rhythm on a rhythm strip, the interval between two consecutive R waves is measured. The distance between succeeding R-R intervals is measured and compared. If the ventricular rhythm is regular, the R-R intervals will measure the same. To evaluate the rhythmicity of the atrial rhythm, the same procedure is used but the interval between two consecutive P waves is measured and compared with succeeding P-P intervals.

SYSTEMATIC RHYTHM INTERPRETATION

A systematic approach to rhythm analysis that is consistently applied when analyzing a rhythm strip is essential (Box 2-1). If you do not develop such an approach, you are more likely to miss something important. Begin analyzing the rhythm strip from left to right.

Box **2-1**	Systematic Rhythm Interpretation

1. Assess rhythmicity (atrial and ventricular).
2. Assess rate (atrial and ventricular).
3. Identify and examine waveforms.
4. Assess intervals (e.g., PR, QRS, QT) and examine ST segments.
5. Interpret the rhythm and assess its clinical significance.

Assess Rhythm/Regularity

The term *rhythm* is used to indicate the site of origin of an electrical impulse (such as a sinus rhythm or ventricular rhythm) and to describe the regularity or irregularity of waveforms. The waveforms on an ECG strip are evaluated for regularity by measuring the distance between the P waves and QRS complexes. If the ventricular rhythm is regular, the R-R intervals will be equal (measure the same). Similarly, if the atrial rhythm is regular, the P-P intervals will be equal. If the variation between the shortest and longest R-R intervals (or P-P intervals) is not exactly the same—but is less than 0.04 second—the rhythm is termed *essentially regular*. If the shortest and longest R-R or P-P intervals vary by more than 0.04 second (one small box), the rhythm is considered *irregular*.

To determine whether the ventricular rhythm is regular or irregular, measure the distance between two consecutive R-R intervals. To determine whether the atrial rhythm is regular or irregular, follow the same procedure previously described for evaluation of ventricular rhythm but measure the distance between two consecutive P-P intervals (instead of R-R intervals) and compare that distance with the other P-P intervals. The P-P intervals will measure the same if the atrial rhythm is regular. For accuracy, the R-R or P-P intervals should be evaluated across an entire 6-second rhythm strip.

Assess Rate

There are several methods used for calculating heart rate. A discussion of each method follows.

Method 1: Six-Second Method

Most ECG paper is printed with 1-second or 3-second markers on the top or bottom of the paper. On ECG paper, 5 large boxes = 1 second, 15 large boxes = 3 seconds, and 30 large boxes = 6 seconds. To determine the ventricular rate, count the number of complete QRS complexes within a period of 6 seconds and multiply that number by 10 to find the number of complexes in 1 minute (Figure 2-14). The 6-second method, also called *the rule of 10*, may be used for regular and irregular rhythms. This is the simplest, quickest, and most commonly used method of rate measurement, but it also is the most inaccurate.

Method 2: Large Boxes

The large box method of rate determination is also called the *rule of 300*. To determine the ventricular rate, count the number of large boxes between an R-R interval and divide into 300 (see Figure 2-14). To determine the atrial rate, count the number of large boxes between a P-P interval and divide into 300 (Table 2-5). This method is best used if the rhythm is regular; however, it may be used if the rhythm is irregular and a rate range (slowest [longest R-R interval] and fastest [shortest R-R interval] rate) is given.

A variation of the large box method is called the *sequence method*. To determine ventricular rate, select an R wave that falls on a dark vertical line. Number the next six consecutive dark vertical lines as follows: 300, 150, 100, 75, 60, and 50 (Figure 2-15). Note where the next R wave falls in relation to the six dark vertical lines already marked. This is the heart rate.

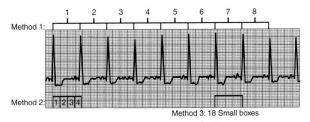

Figure 2-14 Calculating heart rate. Method 1: Number of R-R intervals in 6 seconds × 10 (e.g., 8 × 10 = 80/min). Method 2: Number of large boxes between QRS complexes divided into 300 (e.g., 300 divided by 4 = 75/min). Method 3: Number of small boxes between QRS complexes divided into 1500 (e.g., 1500 divided by 18 = 84/min).

Table **2-5**	Heart Rate Determination Based on the Number of Large Boxes
Number of Large Boxes	**Heart Rate (beats/min)**
1	300
2	150
3	100
4	75
5	60
6	50
7	43
8	38
9	33
10	30

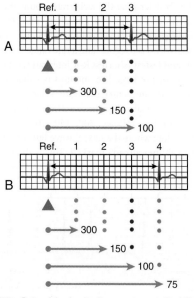

Figure 2-15 Determining heart rate—sequence method. To measure the ventricular rate, find a QRS complex that falls on a heavy dark line. Count 300, 150, 100, 75, 60, and 50 until a second QRS complex occurs. This will be the heart rate. **A,** Heart rate = 100. **B,** Heart rate = 75.

Method 3: Small Boxes

The small box method of rate determination is also called *the rule of 1500*. Each 1-mm box on the graph paper represents 0.04 second. A total of 1500 boxes represents 1 minute (60 sec/min divided by 0.04 sec/box = 1500 boxes/min). To calculate the ventricular rate, count the number of small boxes between the R-R interval and divide into 1500 (see Figure 2-14). To determine the atrial rate, count the number of small boxes between the P-P interval and divide into 1500. This method is time consuming but accurate. If the rhythm is irregular, a rate range should be given.

Identify and Examine Waveforms

Look to see whether the normal waveforms (P, Q, R, S, and T) are present. To locate P waves, look to the left of each QRS complex. Normally, one P wave precedes each QRS complex; they occur regularly (P-P intervals are equal), and they look similar in size, shape, and position.

Next, evaluate the QRS complex. Are QRS complexes present? If so, does a QRS follow each P wave? Do the QRS complexes look alike? Assess the T waves. Does a T wave follow each QRS complex? Does a P wave follow the T wave? Are the T waves upright and of normal height? Look to see whether a U wave is present. If so, note its height and direction (positive or negative).

Assess Intervals and Examine Segments

PR Interval

Intervals are measured to evaluate conduction. Is a PRI present? If so, measure the PRI and determine whether they are equal. The PRI is measured from the point where the P wave leaves the baseline to the beginning of the QRS complex. Are the PRIs within normal limits? Remember that a normal PRI measures 0.12 to 0.20 second. If the PRIs are the same, they are said to be constant. If the PRIs are different, is a pattern present? In some dysrhythmias, the duration of the PRI will increase until a P wave appears with no QRS after it. This is referred to as *lengthening* of the PRI. PRIs that vary in duration and have no pattern are said to be *variable*.

QRS Duration

Identify the QRS complexes and measure their duration. The beginning of the QRS is measured from the point at which the first wave of the complex begins to deviate from the baseline. The point at which the last wave of the complex begins to level out at, above, or below the baseline marks the end of the QRS complex. The QRS is considered narrow (i.e., normal) if it measures 0.11 second or less and is considered wide if it measures more than 0.11 second. A narrow QRS complex is presumed to be supraventricular in origin.

QT Interval

To determine the QT interval, measure the interval between two consecutive R waves (R-R interval). If the measured QT interval is less than half the R-R interval of that QRS complex and the R wave of the following complex, it is probably normal (provided the patient's heart rate is 95 beats/min or less). Alternately, count the number of small boxes between the beginning of the QRS complex and the end of the T wave. Then multiply that number by 0.04 second. If no Q wave is present, measure the QT interval from the beginning of the R wave to the end of the T wave. In general, a QT interval of 0.44 second or less is considered normal.

Examine ST Segments

Determine the presence of ST-segment elevation or depression. Remember that the TP segment is used as the baseline from which to evaluate the degree of displacement of the ST segment from the isoelectric line. If ST-segment displacement is present, note the number of millimeters of deviation from the isoelectric line or from the patient's baseline at a point 0.06 or 0.08 second after the J point.

Interpret the Rhythm

Interpret the rhythm, specifying the site of origin (pacemaker site) of the rhythm (sinus), the mechanism (bradycardia), and the ventricular rate. For example, "Sinus bradycardia at 38 beats/min." Assess the patient to find out how he or she is tolerating the rate and rhythm.

Sinus Mechanisms

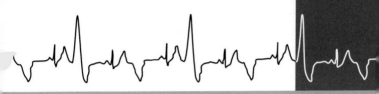

The normal heartbeat is the result of an electrical impulse that starts in the sinoatrial (SA) node. Normally, pacemaker cells within the SA node spontaneously depolarize more rapidly than other cardiac cells. As a result, the SA node usually dominates other areas that may be depolarizing at a slightly slower rate. The impulse is sent to cells at the outside edge of the SA node and then to the myocardial cells of the surrounding atrium.

A rhythm that begins in the SA node has the following characteristics:

- A positive (i.e., upright) P wave before each QRS complex
- P waves that look alike
- A constant PR interval
- A regular atrial and ventricular rhythm (usually)

SINUS RHYTHM

Sinus rhythm is the name given to a normal heart rhythm. Sinus rhythm is sometimes called a *regular sinus rhythm* (RSR) or *normal sinus rhythm* (NSR). Sinus rhythm reflects normal electrical activity—that is, the rhythm starts in the SA node and then heads down the normal conduction pathway through the atria, atrioventricular (AV) node and bundle, right and left bundle branches, and Purkinje fibers. In adults and adolescents, the SA node normally fires at a regular rate of 60 to 100 beats/min. Figure 3-1 shows an example of a sinus rhythm recorded simultaneously in three leads: V_1, II, and V_5. A summary of the electrocardiogram (ECG) characteristics of a sinus rhythm is shown in Table 3-1.

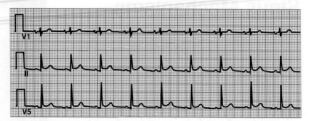

Figure 3-1   Sinus rhythm at 80 beats/min, ST-segment elevation.

Table **3-1**	Characteristics of Sinus Rhythm
Rhythm	R-R and P-P intervals are regular
Rate	60 to 100 beats/min
P waves	Positive (upright) in lead II; one precedes each QRS complex; P waves look alike
PR interval	0.12 to 0.20 sec and constant from beat to beat
QRS duration	0.11 sec or less unless abnormally conducted

SINUS BRADYCARDIA

If the SA node fires at a rate that is slower than normal for the patient's age, the rhythm is called *sinus bradycardia*. The rhythm starts in the SA node and then travels the normal conduction pathway, resulting in atrial and ventricular depolarization. In adults and adolescents, a sinus bradycardia has a heart rate of less than 60 beats/min. The term *severe sinus bradycardia* is sometimes used to describe a sinus bradycardia with a rate of less than 40 beats/min.

If a patient presents with a bradycardia, assess how the patient is tolerating the rhythm at rest and with activity. If the patient has no symptoms, no treatment is necessary. The term *symptomatic bradycardia* is used to describe a patient who experiences signs and symptoms of hemodynamic compromise related to a slow heart rate. Treatment of a symptomatic bradycardia should include assessment of the patient's oxygen saturation level and determining whether signs of increased work of breathing are present (e.g., retractions, tachypnea, paradoxic abdominal breathing). Give supplemental oxygen if

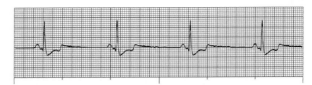

Figure 3-2   Sinus bradycardia at 40 beats/min with ST-segment depression and inverted T waves.

Table **3-2**	Characteristics of Sinus Bradycardia
Rhythm	R-R and P-P intervals are regular
Rate	Less than 60 beats/min
P waves	Positive (upright) in lead II; one precedes each QRS complex; P waves look alike
PR interval	0.12 to 0.20 sec and constant from beat to beat
QRS duration	0.11 sec or less unless abnormally conducted

oxygenation is inadequate and assist breathing if ventilation is inadequate. Establish intravenous (IV) access and obtain a 12-lead ECG. Atropine, administered intravenously, is the drug of choice for symptomatic bradycardia. Reassess the patient's response and continue monitoring the patient. An example of sinus bradycardia is shown in Figure 3-2. The ECG characteristics of sinus bradycardia are shown in Table 3-2.

SINUS TACHYCARDIA

If the SA node fires at a rate faster than normal for the patient's age, the rhythm is called *sinus tachycardia*. Sinus tachycardia begins and ends gradually. Treatment for sinus tachycardia is directed at correcting the underlying cause (i.e., fluid replacement, relief of pain, removal of offending medications or substances, reducing fever or anxiety). Sinus tachycardia in a patient experiencing an acute myocardial infarction (MI) may be treated with medications to slow the heart rate and decrease myocardial oxygen demand (e.g., beta-blockers), provided there are no signs of heart failure or other contraindications. An example of sinus tachycardia is shown in Figure 3-3. The ECG characteristics of sinus tachycardia appear in Table 3-3.

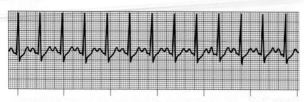

Figure 3-3   Sinus tachycardia at 125 beats/min with ST-segment depression.

Table **3-3**	Characteristics of Sinus Tachycardia
Rhythm	R-R and P-P intervals are regular
Rate	101 to 180 beats/min
P waves	Positive (upright) in lead II; one precedes each QRS complex; P waves look alike
PR interval	0.12 to 0.20 sec and constant from beat to beat
QRS duration	0.11 sec or less unless abnormally conducted

SINUS ARRHYTHMIA

When the SA node fires irregularly, the resulting rhythm is called *sinus arrhythmia*. Sinus arrhythmia that is associated with the phases of breathing and changes in intrathoracic pressure is called *respiratory sinus arrhythmia*. Sinus arrhythmia that is not related to the respiratory cycle is called *nonrespiratory sinus arrhythmia*. Sinus arrhythmia usually does not require treatment unless it is accompanied by a slow heart rate that causes hemodynamic compromise. If hemodynamic compromise is present as a result of the slow rate, IV atropine may be indicated to treat the bradycardia. An example of sinus arrhythmia is shown in Figure 3-4. The characteristics of sinus arrhythmia are shown in Table 3-4.

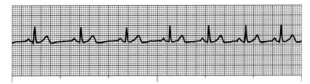

Figure 3-4 Sinus arrhythmia at 63 to 81 beats/min.

Table **3-4**	Characteristics of Sinus Arrhythmia
Rhythm	Irregular and phasic with breathing; heart rate increases gradually during inspiration (R-R intervals shorten) and decreases with expiration (R-R intervals lengthen)
Rate	Usually 60 to 100 beats/min, but may be slower or faster
P waves	Positive (upright) in lead II; one precedes each QRS complex; P waves look alike
PR interval	0.12 to 0.20 sec and constant from beat to beat
QRS duration	0.11 sec or less unless abnormally conducted

SINOATRIAL BLOCK

With SA block, which is also called *sinus exit block*, the pacemaker cells within the SA node initiate an impulse but it is blocked as it exits the SA node. This results in periodically absent PQRST complexes. SA block is thought to occur because of failure of the transitional cells in the SA node to conduct the impulse from the pacemaker cells to the surrounding atrium.

Signs and symptoms associated with SA block depend on the number of sinus beats blocked. If the episodes of SA block are transient and there are no significant signs or symptoms, the patient is observed. If signs of hemodynamic compromise are present and are the result of medication toxicity, the offending agents should be withheld. If the episodes of SA block are frequent, IV atropine, temporary pacing, or insertion of a permanent pacemaker may be needed. An example of SA block is shown in Figure 3-5. The ECG characteristics of SA block appear in Table 3-5.

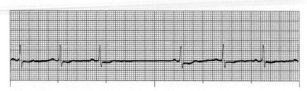

Figure 3-5 Sinus rhythm at a rate of 36 to 71 beats/min with an episode of sinoatrial (SA) block.

Table **3-5**	Characteristics of Sinoatrial Block
Rhythm	Irregular as a result of the pause(s) caused by the SA block—the pause is the same as, or an exact multiple of, the distance between two other P-P intervals
Rate	Usually normal but varies because of the pause
P waves	Positive (i.e., upright) in lead II; P waves look alike; when present, one precedes each QRS complex.
PR interval	0.12 to 0.20 sec and constant from beat to beat
QRS duration	0.11 sec or less unless abnormally conducted

SINUS ARREST

With sinus arrest, the pacemaker cells of the SA node fail to initiate an electrical impulse for one or more beats, resulting in absent PQRST complexes on the ECG. When the SA node fails to initiate an impulse, an escape pacemaker site (e.g., the AV junction or the Purkinje fibers) should assume responsibility for pacing the heart. If an escape pacemaker site does not fire, you will see absent PQRST complexes on the ECG.

If the episodes of sinus arrest are transient and there are no significant signs or symptoms, observe the patient. If hemodynamic compromise is present, IV atropine, temporary pacing, or both may be indicated. If the episodes of sinus arrest are frequent and prolonged (i.e., more than 3 seconds) or a result of disease of the SA node, insertion of a permanent pacemaker is generally warranted. An example of sinus arrest is shown in Figure 3-6. The ECG characteristics of sinus arrest are shown in Table 3-6.

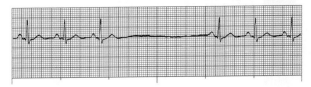

Figure 3-6   Sinus rhythm at a rate of 24 to 81 beats/min with an episode of sinus arrest.

Table **3-6**	**Characteristics of Sinus Arrest**
Rhythm	Irregular; the pause is of undetermined length, more than one PQRST complex is missing, and it is not the same distance as other P-P intervals
Rate	Usually normal but varies because of the pause
P waves	Positive (i.e., upright) in lead II; P waves look alike; when present, one precedes each QRS complex
PR interval	0.12 to 0.20 sec and constant from beat to beat
QRS duration	0.11 sec or less unless abnormally conducted

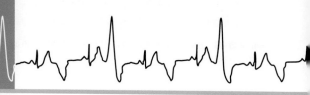

P waves reflect atrial depolarization. A rhythm that begins in the sinoatrial (SA) node has one positive (i.e., upright) P wave before each QRS complex. A rhythm that begins in the atria will have a positive P wave that is shaped differently from P waves that begin in the SA node. This difference in P wave configuration occurs because the impulse begins in the atria and follows a different conduction pathway to the atrioventricular (AV) node.

PREMATURE ATRIAL COMPLEXES

A *premature atrial complex* (PAC) occurs when an irritable site (i.e., focus) within the atria fires before the next SA node impulse is expected to fire (Figure 4-1). This interrupts the sinus rhythm. If the irritable site is close to the SA node, the atrial P wave will look very similar to the P waves initiated by the SA node. The P wave of a PAC may be biphasic (i.e., partly positive, partly negative); flattened; notched; pointed; or lost in the preceding T wave. PACs usually do not require treatment if they are infrequent. The patient may complain of a "skipped beat" or occasional "palpitations" if PACs are frequent or may be unaware of their occurrence. In susceptible individuals, frequent PACs may induce episodes of atrial fibrillation or paroxysmal supraventricular tachycardia (PSVT). Frequent PACs are treated by correcting the underlying cause. If the patient is symptomatic, frequent PACs may be treated with beta-blockers. The electrocardiogram (ECG) characteristics of PACs are shown in Table 4-1.

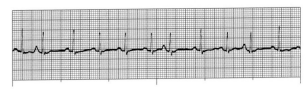

Figure 4-1 Sinus tachycardia with three PACs. From the left, beats 2, 7, and 10 are PACs.

Table **4-1**	Characteristics of Premature Atrial Complexes
Rhythm	Regular with premature beats
Rate	Usually within normal range, but depends on underlying rhythm
P waves	Premature (occurring earlier than the next expected sinus P wave), positive (upright) in lead II, one before each QRS complex, often differ in shape from sinus P waves—may be flattened, notched, pointed, biphasic, or lost in the preceding T wave
PR interval	May be normal or prolonged depending on the prematurity of the beat
QRS duration	Usually 0.11 sec or less but may be wide (aberrant) or absent, depending on the prematurity of the beat; the QRS of the PAC is similar in shape to those of the underlying rhythm unless the PAC is abnormally conducted

Aberrantly Conducted Premature Atrial Complexes

PACs associated with a wide QRS complex are called *aberrantly conducted PACs*. This indicates that conduction through the ventricles is abnormal (Figure 4-2).

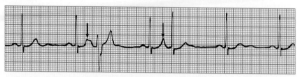

Aberrantly conducted PAC PAC conducted normally

Figure 4-2   Premature atrial complexes (PACs) with and without abnormal conduction (aberrancy).

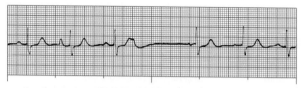

Figure 4-3   Sinus rhythm with a nonconducted (blocked) PAC. Note the distorted T wave of the third QRS complex from the left.

Nonconducted Premature Atrial Complexes

Sometimes, when a PAC occurs very early and close to the T wave of the preceding beat, only a P wave may be seen with no QRS after it (appearing as a pause) (Figure 4-3). This type of PAC is called a *nonconducted* or *blocked* PAC because the P wave occurred too early to be conducted.

WANDERING ATRIAL PACEMAKER

Multiformed atrial rhythm is an updated term for the rhythm formerly known as *wandering atrial pacemaker*. With this rhythm, the size, shape, and direction of the P waves vary, sometimes from beat to beat. The difference in the look of the P waves is a result of the gradual shifting of the dominant pacemaker among the SA node, the atria, and the AV junction (Figure 4-4).

Wandering atrial pacemaker is usually a transient rhythm that resolves on its own when the firing rate of the SA node increases and the sinus resumes pacing responsibility. If the rhythm occurs because of digitalis toxicity, the drug should be withheld. The ECG characteristics of wandering atrial pacemaker are shown in Table 4-2.

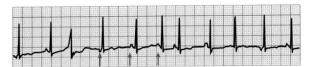

Figure 4-4 Wandering atrial pacemaker. Note the differences in the shapes of the P waves.

Table **4-2**	Characteristics of Wandering Atrial Pacemaker
Rhythm	Usually irregular as the pacemaker site shifts from the SA node to ectopic atrial locations or AV junction
Rate	Usually 60 to 100 beats/min, but may be slower; if the rate is faster than 100 beats/min, the rhythm is termed *multifocal* (or *chaotic*) *atrial tachycardia*
P waves	Size, shape, and direction may change from beat to beat; may be upright, inverted, biphasic, rounded, flat, pointed, notched, or buried in the QRS complex
PR interval	Varies as the pacemaker site shifts from the SA node to ectopic atrial locations or AV junction
QRS duration	0.11 sec or less unless abnormally conducted

MULTIFOCAL ATRIAL TACHYCARDIA

When the wandering atrial pacemaker rhythm is associated with a ventricular rate of more than 100 beats/min, the dysrhythmia is called *multifocal atrial tachycardia* (MAT) or *chaotic atrial tachycardia* (Figure 4-5). In MAT, multiple ectopic sites stimulate the atria. MAT may be confused with atrial fibrillation because both rhythms are irregular; however, P waves, although varying in size, shape, and direction, are clearly visible in MAT. The treatment of MAT is directed at the underlying cause. If you know the rhythm is MAT and the patient is symptomatic, it is best to consult a cardiologist before starting treatment. If the

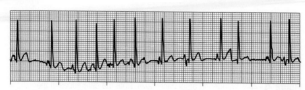

Figure 4-5   Multifocal atrial tachycardia (MAT), also known as *chaotic atrial tachycardia.*

patient is stable but symptomatic and you are uncertain that the rhythm is MAT, you can try a vagal maneuver. If vagal maneuvers are ineffective, intravenous (IV) adenosine can be tried. Remember that MAT is the result of the random and chaotic firing of multiple sites in the atria; MAT does not involve reentry through the AV node. Therefore, it is unlikely that vagal maneuvers or giving adenosine will terminate the rhythm; however, they may momentarily slow the rate enough so that you can look at the P waves and determine the specific type of tachycardia. By determining the type of tachycardia, treatment specific to that rhythm can be given. The ECG characteristics of MAT are shown in Table 4-3.

Table **4-3**	Characteristics of Multifocal Atrial Tachycardia
Rhythm	Usually irregular as the pacemaker site shifts from the SA node to ectopic atrial locations or AV junction
Rate	Faster than 100 beats/min
P waves	Size, shape, and direction may change from beat to beat; may be upright, inverted, biphasic, rounded, flat, pointed, notched, or buried in the QRS complex
PR interval	Varies as the pacemaker site shifts from the SA node to ectopic atrial locations or AV junction
QRS duration	0.11 sec or less unless abnormally conducted

SUPRAVENTRICULAR TACHYCARDIA

Supraventricular arrhythmias begin above the bifurcation of the bundle of His. This means that supraventricular arrhythmias include rhythms that begin in the SA node, atrial tissue, or the AV junction. The term *supraventricular tachycardia* (SVT) includes three main types of fast rhythms, which are shown in Figure 4-6.

- Atrial tachycardia (AT). During AT, an irritable site in the atria fires automatically at a rapid rate.
- Atrioventricular nodal reentrant tachycardia (AVNRT), which is also called *AV nodal reciprocating tachycardia*. During AVNRT, fast and slow pathways in the AV node form an electrical circuit or loop. The impulse moves in a repeating loop around the AV nodal (junctional) area.
- Atrioventricular reentrant tachycardia (AVRT), which is also called *AV reciprocating tachycardia*. During AVRT, the impulse begins above the ventricles but travels by means of a pathway other than the AV node and bundle of His.

ATRIAL TACHYCARDIA

AT consists of a series of rapid beats from an irritable site in the atria (Figure 4-7). This rapid atrial rate overrides the SA node and becomes the pacemaker. Conduction of the atrial impulse to the ventricles is often 1:1. This means that every atrial impulse is conducted through the AV node to the ventricles. This results in a P wave preceding each QRS complex. Although the P waves appear upright, they tend to look different from those seen when the impulse is initiated from the SA node. Because conducted impulses travel through the ventricles in the usual manner, the QRS complexes appear normal.

The term *paroxysmal* is used to describe a rhythm that starts or ends suddenly. AT that starts or ends suddenly is called *paroxysmal supraventricular tachycardia* (PSVT), once called *paroxysmal atrial tachycardia* (PAT) (Figure 4-8). With very rapid atrial rates, the AV node begins to filter some of the

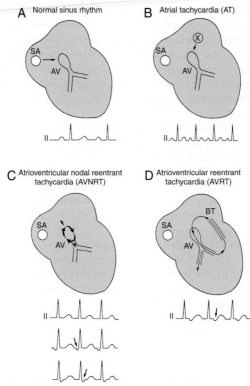

Figure 4-6   Types of supraventricular tachycardias. **A,** Normal sinus rhythm is shown here as a reference. **B,** With AT, a focus (X) outside the SA node fires off automatically at a rapid rate. **C,** With AVNRT, the cardiac stimulus originates as a wave of excitation that spins around the AV junctional area. As a result, P waves may be buried in the QRS or appear immediately before or just after the QRS complex *(arrows)* because of nearly simultaneous activation of the atria and ventricles. **D,** A similar type of reentrant (circus movement) mechanism in Wolff-Parkinson-White syndrome. This mechanism is referred to as atrioventricular reentrant tachycardia (AVRT). Note the P wave in lead II somewhat after the QRS complex.

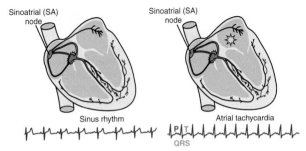

Figure 4-7 Atrial tachycardia. AV, atrioventricular; SA, sinoatrial.

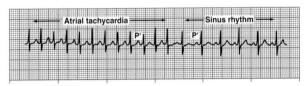

Figure 4-8 Paroxysmal supraventricular tachycardia that ends spontaneously with the abrupt resumption of sinus rhythm. The P waves of the tachycardia (rate: about 150 beats/min) are superimposed on the preceding T waves.

impulses coming to it. By doing so it protects the ventricles from excessively rapid rates. When the AV node selectively filters conduction of some of these impulses, the rhythm is called *paroxysmal supraventricular tachycardia with block*.

If episodes of AT are short, the patient may be asymptomatic. A rhythm that lasts from three beats up to 30 seconds is a *nonsustained rhythm*. A *sustained rhythm* is one that lasts more than 30 seconds. If AT is sustained and the patient is symptomatic as a result of the rapid rate, treatment should include applying a pulse oximeter and administering oxygen (if indicated), obtaining the patient's vital signs, and establishing IV access. A 12-lead ECG should be obtained. If the

Table **4-4**	Characteristics of Atrial Tachycardia
Rhythm	Regular
Rate	150 to 250 beats/min
P waves	One P wave precedes each QRS complex in lead II; these P waves differ in shape from sinus P waves; an isoelectric baseline is usually present between P waves; if the atrial rhythm originates in the low portion of the atrium, P waves will be negative in lead II; with rapid rates, it may be difficult to distinguish P waves from T waves.
PR interval	May be shorter or longer than normal; may be difficult to measure because P waves may be hidden in the T waves of preceding beats
QRS duration	0.11 sec or less unless abnormally conducted

patient is not hypotensive, vagal maneuvers may be tried. Although AT will rarely stop with vagal maneuvers, they are used to try to stop the rhythm or slow conduction through the AV node. If vagal maneuvers fail, antiarrhythmic medications should be tried. Adenosine is the drug of choice, except in patients with severe asthma. If needed, calcium channel blockers or beta-blockers may be used to slow the ventricular rate. If AT is sustained and causing persistent signs of hemodynamic compromise, synchronized cardioversion should be performed. The ECG characteristics of AT are shown in Table 4-4.

ATRIOVENTRICULAR NODAL REENTRANT TACHYCARDIA

AVNRT is the most common type of SVT. It is caused by reentry in the area of the AV node. In the normal AV node, there is only one pathway through which an electrical impulse is conducted from the SA node to the ventricles. Patients with AVNRT have two conduction pathways within the AV node that conduct impulses at different speeds and recover at different rates. Under the right conditions, these pathways can form an electrical circuit or loop. As one side of the loop is recovering, the other is firing.

AVNRT is usually caused by a PAC that is spread by the electrical circuit. This allows the impulse to spin around in a circle indefinitely and to reenter the normal electrical pathway with each pass around the circuit. The result is a very rapid and regular ventricular rhythm that ranges from 150 to 250 beats/min (Figure 4-9).

Because AVNRT may be short-lived or sustained, treatment depends on the duration of the tachycardia and severity of the patient's signs and symptoms. If the patient is stable but symptomatic and the symptoms are the result of the rapid heart rate, apply a pulse oximeter and administer supplemental oxygen, if indicated. Obtain the patient's vital signs, establish IV access, and obtain a 12-lead ECG. While continuously monitoring the patient's ECG, attempt a vagal maneuver if there are no contraindications. If vagal maneuvers do not slow the rate or cause conversion of the tachycardia to a sinus rhythm, the first antiarrhythmic given is adenosine. If the patient is unstable, treatment should include application of a pulse oximeter and administration of supplemental oxygen (if indicated), IV access, and sedation (if the patient is awake and time permits), followed by synchronized cardioversion.

The ECG characteristics of AVNRT are summarized in Table 4-5.

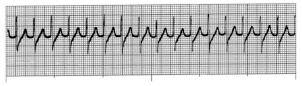

Figure 4-9   Atrioventricular nodal reentrant tachycardia (AVNRT).

Table **4-5**	Characteristics of Atrioventricular Nodal Reentrant Tachycardia
Rhythm	Ventricular rhythm is usually very regular
Rate	150 to 250 beats/min; typically 180 to 200 beats/min in adults
P waves	P waves are often hidden in the QRS complex; if the ventricles are stimulated first and then the atria, a negative (inverted) P wave will appear after the QRS in leads II, III, and aVF; when the atria are depolarized after the ventricles, the P wave typically distorts the end of the QRS complex.
PR interval	P waves are not seen before the QRS complex; therefore, the PR interval is not measurable
QRS duration	0.11 sec or less unless abnormally conducted

ATRIOVENTRICULAR REENTRANT TACHYCARDIA

The next most common type of SVT is AVRT. Remember that the AV node is normally the only electrical connection between the atria and the ventricles. AVRT involves a pathway of impulse conduction outside the AV node and the bundle of His. The term *preexcitation* is used to describe rhythms that originate from above the ventricles but in which the impulse travels via a pathway other than the AV node and the AV bundle. As a result, the supraventricular impulse excites the ventricles earlier than would be expected if the impulse traveled by way of the normal conduction system. Patients with preexcitation syndromes are prone to AVRT. The most common type of preexcitation syndrome is called *Wolff-Parkinson-White (WPW) syndrome*.

When WPW is associated with a sinus rhythm, the P wave looks normal. Remember that the AV node normally delays the impulse it receives from the SA node. The delay in conduction allows the atria to empty blood into the ventricles before the next ventricular contraction begins. In WPW, the PR interval is short (less than 0.12 second) because the impulse travels very quickly across the accessory pathway, bypassing the normal delay in the AV node (Figure 4-10). As the impulse crosses the insertion point of the accessory pathway in the ventricular muscle, that part of the

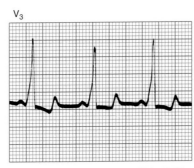

Figure 4-10 Lead V₃. Typical Wolff-Parkinson-White (WPW) pattern showing the short PR interval, delta wave, wide QRS complex, and secondary ST-segment and T-wave changes.

ventricle is stimulated earlier (preexcited) than if the impulse had followed the normal conduction pathway through the bundle of His and Purkinje fibers. On the ECG, preexcitation of the ventricles can be seen as a *delta wave* in some leads. A delta wave is an initial slurred deflection at the beginning of the QRS complex that may be positive or negative and reflects the abnormal depolarization of the ventricles through the accessory pathway.

Consultation with a cardiologist is recommended when caring for a patient with AVRT. The ECG characteristics of WPW are summarized in Table 4-6.

Table **4-6**	Characteristics of Wolff-Parkinson-White Syndrome
Rhythm	Regular, unless associated with atrial fibrillation
Rate	Usually 60 to 100 beats/min, if the underlying rhythm is sinus in origin
P waves	Normal and positive in lead II unless WPW syndrome is associated with atrial fibrillation
PR interval	If P waves are observed, 0.12 sec or less, because the impulse travels very quickly across the accessory pathway, bypassing the normal delay in the atrioventricular (AV) node
QRS duration	Usually more than 0.12 sec; slurred upstroke of the QRS complex (delta wave) may be seen in one or more leads.

ATRIAL FLUTTER

Atrial flutter is an ectopic atrial rhythm in which an irritable site within the atria fires regularly at a very rapid rate (Figure 4-11). Atrial flutter has been classified into two types.

- Type I atrial flutter, which is also called *typical atrial flutter*, is caused by reentry. In this type of atrial flutter, an impulse circles around a large area of tissue, such as the entire right atrium. The atrial rate ranges from 250 to 350 beats/min.
- Type II atrial flutter is also called *atypical* or *very rapid atrial flutter*. The precise mechanism of type II atrial flutter has not been defined. Patients with this type of atrial flutter often develop atrial fibrillation. In type II atrial flutter, the atrial rate ranges from 350 to 450 beats/min.

It is best to consult a cardiologist when considering treatment options. If atrial flutter is associated with a rapid ventricular rate and the patient is stable but symptomatic, treatment is usually aimed at controlling the ventricular rate with medications such as diltiazem or beta-blockers. Beta-blockers should generally be avoided in the presence of severe underlying pulmonary disease or heart failure. Synchronized cardioversion should be considered for any patient with atrial flutter who has serious signs and symptoms because of the rapid ventricular rate. The ECG characteristics of atrial flutter are shown in Table 4-7.

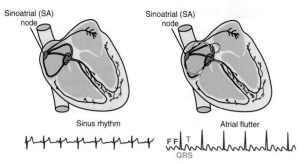

Figure 4-11   Atrial flutter. F, flutter wave.

Table 4-7	Characteristics of Atrial Flutter
Rhythm	Atrial regular; ventricular regular or irregular depending on AV conduction and blockade
Rate	With type I atrial flutter, the atrial rate ranges from 250 to 350 beats/min; with type II atrial flutter, the atrial rate ranges from 350 to 450 beats/min; the ventricular rate varies and is determined by AV blockade; the ventricular rate will usually not exceed 180 beats/min as a result of the intrinsic conduction rate of the AV junction
P waves	No identifiable P waves; saw-toothed "flutter" waves are present
PR interval	Not measurable
QRS duration	0.11 sec or less but may be widened if flutter waves are buried in the QRS complex or if abnormally conducted

ATRIAL FIBRILLATION

Atrial fibrillation (AFib) occurs because of irritable sites in the atria firing at a rate of 400 to 600 times/min. These rapid impulses cause the muscles of the atria to quiver (i.e., fibrillate), thereby resulting in ineffectual atrial contraction, decreased stroke volume, a subsequent decrease in cardiac output, and a loss of atrial kick.

Treatment decisions are based on the ventricular rate, the duration of the rhythm, the patient's general health, and how he or she tolerates the rhythm. It is best to consult a cardiologist when considering specific therapies. The two primary treatment strategies used to control symptoms associated with AFib are rate control and rhythm control. With rate control, the patient remains in AFib but the ventricular rate is controlled to decrease acute symptoms, reduce signs of ischemia, and reduce or prevent signs of heart failure from developing. With rhythm control, sinus rhythm is reestablished.

If AFib is associated with a rapid ventricular rate and the patient is stable but symptomatic, treatment is usually aimed at controlling the ventricular rate with medications such as diltiazem, which is a calcium channel blocker, or beta-blockers. Synchronized cardioversion should be considered if the patient with AFib has serious signs and symptoms because of the rapid ventricular rate. An example of AFib is shown in Figure 4-12 and its ECG characteristics appear in Table 4-8.

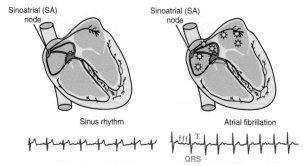

Figure 4-12   Atrial fibrillation. AV, atrioventricular; f, fibrillatory wave.

Table **4-8**	Characteristics of Atrial Fibrillation
Rhythm	Ventricular rhythm usually irregularly irregular
Rate	Atrial rate usually 400 to 600 beats/min; ventricular rate variable
P waves	No identifiable P waves, fibrillatory waves present; erratic, wavy baseline
PR interval	Not measurable
QRS duration	0.11 sec or less unless abnormally conducted

Junctional Rhythms

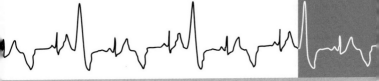

If the atrioventricular (AV) junction paces the heart, the electrical impulse must travel in a backward (*retrograde*) direction to activate the atria (Figure 5-1). If a P wave is seen, it will be inverted in leads II, III, and aVF because the impulse is traveling away from the positive electrode. The QRS duration associated with a rhythm that begins in the AV junction measures 0.11 second or less if conduction through the bundle branches, Purkinje fibers, and ventricles is normal.

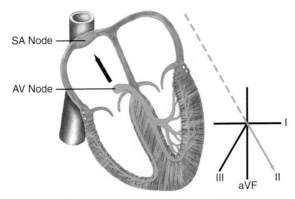

Figure 5-1 If the AV junction paces the heart, the electrical impulse must travel in a backward (retrograde) direction to activate the atria. SA, sinoatrial.

PREMATURE JUNCTIONAL COMPLEXES

A *premature junctional complex* (PJC) occurs when an irritable site within the AV junction fires before the next sinoatrial (SA) node impulse is ready to fire. This interrupts the sinus rhythm. Because the impulse is conducted through the ventricles in the usual manner, the QRS complex will usually measure 0.11 second or less.

PJCs do not normally require treatment because most individuals who have PJCs are asymptomatic. If PJCs occur because of ingestion of stimulants or digitalis toxicity, these substances should be withheld. Examples of PJCs are shown in Figure 5-2. The electrocardiogram (ECG) characteristics of PJCs are shown in Table 5-1.

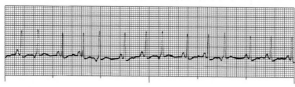

Figure 5-2 Sinus tachycardia at 136 beats/min with frequent PJCs.

Table **5-1**	Characteristics of Premature Junctional Complexes
Rhythm	Regular with *premature* beats
Rate	Usually within normal range, but depends on underlying rhythm
P waves	May occur before, during, or after the QRS; if visible, the P wave is inverted in leads II, III, and aVF
PR interval	If a P wave occurs before the QRS, the PR interval will usually be 0.12 sec or less; if no P wave occurs before the QRS, there will be no PR interval
QRS duration	0.11 sec or less unless abnormally conducted

JUNCTIONAL ESCAPE BEATS/RHYTHM

A junctional escape beat begins in the AV junction and appears *late* (after the next expected sinus beat. Junctional escape beats frequently occur during episodes of sinus arrest or they follow pauses of nonconducted premature atrial complexes (PACs). An example of a junctional escape beat is shown in Figure 5-3. The ECG characteristics of junctional escape beats are summarized in Table 5-2.

A junctional *rhythm* is several sequential junctional escape *beats.* The terms *junctional rhythm* and *junctional escape rhythm* are used interchangeably. Remember that the intrinsic rate of the AV junction is 40 to 60 beats/min. Because a junctional rhythm starts from above the ventricles, the QRS complex is usually narrow and its rhythm is very regular. Treatment depends on the cause of the dysrhythmia and the patient's presenting signs and

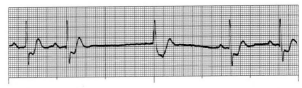

Figure 5-3 Sinus rhythm at 71 beats/min with a prolonged PR interval (0.24 sec), an episode of sinus arrest, a junctional escape beat, and ST-segment depression.

Table **5-2**	Characteristics of Junctional Escape Beats
Rhythm	Regular with *late* beats
Rate	Usually within normal range, but depends on underlying rhythm
P waves	May occur before, during, or after the QRS; if visible, the P wave is inverted in leads II, III, and aVF
PR interval	If a P wave occurs before the QRS, the PR interval will usually be 0.12 sec or less; if no P wave occurs before the QRS, there will be no PR interval
QRS duration	0.11 sec or less unless abnormally conducted

symptoms. If the dysrhythmia is caused by digitalis toxicity, this medication should be withheld. If the patient's signs and symptoms are related to the slow heart rate, treatment should include application of a pulse oximeter and administration of supplemental oxygen, if indicated. Establish intravenous (IV) access, obtain a 12-lead ECG, and administer IV atropine. Reassess the patient's response and continue monitoring the patient. An example of a junctional rhythm is shown in Figure 5-4. The ECG characteristics of a junctional rhythm are shown in Table 5-3.

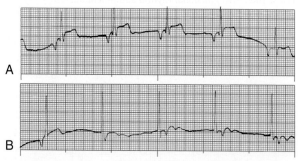

Figure 5-4   Junctional escape rhythm. Continuous strips. **A,** Note the inverted (retrograde) P waves before the QRS complexes. **B,** Note the change in the location of the P waves. In the first beat, the retrograde P wave is seen before the QRS. In the second beat, no P wave is seen. In the remaining beats, the P wave is seen after the QRS complexes.

Table **5-3**	Characteristics of Junctional Escape Rhythm
Rhythm	Very regular
Rate	40 to 60 beats/min
P waves	May occur before, during, or after the QRS; if visible, the P wave is inverted in leads II, III, and aVF
PR interval	If a P wave occurs before the QRS, the PR interval will usually be 0.12 sec or less; if no P wave occurs before the QRS, there will be no PR interval
QRS duration	0.11 sec or less unless abnormally conducted

ACCELERATED JUNCTIONAL RHYTHM

If the AV junction speeds up and fires at a rate of 61 to 100 beats/min, the resulting rhythm is called an *accelerated junctional rhythm*. The only ECG difference between a junctional rhythm and an accelerated junctional rhythm is the increase in the ventricular rate. The patient is usually asymptomatic because the ventricular rate is 61 to 100 beats/min; however, the patient should be monitored closely. If the rhythm is caused by digitalis toxicity, this medication should be withheld. An example of an accelerated junctional rhythm is shown in Figure 5-5. The ECG characteristics of this rhythm are shown in Table 5-4.

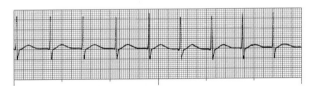

Figure 5-5   Accelerated junctional rhythm at 93 beats/min.

Table **5-4**	Characteristics of Accelerated Junctional Rhythm
Rhythm	Very regular
Rate	61 to 100 beats/min
P waves	May occur before, during, or after the QRS; if visible, the P wave is inverted in leads II, III, and aVF
PR interval	If a P wave occurs before the QRS, the PR interval will usually be 0.12 sec or less; if no P wave occurs before the QRS, there will be no PR interval
QRS duration	0.11 sec or less unless abnormally conducted

JUNCTIONAL TACHYCARDIA

Junctional tachycardia is an ectopic rhythm that begins in the pacemaker cells found in the bundle of His. When three or more sequential PJCs occur at a rate of more than 100 beats/min, a junctional tachycardia exists. *Nonparoxysmal* (i.e., gradual onset) *junctional tachycardia* usually starts as an accelerated junctional rhythm, but the heart rate gradually increases to more than 100 beats/min. The usual ventricular rate for nonparoxysmal junctional tachycardia is 101 to 140 beats/min. *Paroxysmal junctional tachycardia*, which is also known as *focal* or *automatic junctional tachycardia*, is an uncommon dysrhythmia that starts and ends suddenly and is often precipitated by a PJC. The ventricular rate for paroxysmal junctional tachycardia is generally faster, at a rate of 140 beats/min or more. When the ventricular rate is greater than 150 beats/min, it is difficult to distinguish junctional tachycardia from atrioventricular nodal reentrant tachycardia (AVNRT) and atrioventricular reentrant tachycardia (AVRT).

Treatment depends on the severity of the patient's signs and symptoms, and expert consultation is advised. If the patient is symptomatic because of the rapid rate, initial treatment should include application of a pulse oximeter and administration of supplemental oxygen, if indicated. Establish IV access and obtain a 12-lead ECG. Because it is often difficult to distinguish junctional tachycardia from other narrow-QRS tachycardias, vagal maneuvers and, if necessary, IV adenosine may be used to help determine the origin of the rhythm. A beta-blocker or calcium channel blocker may be ordered (if no contraindications exist) to slow conduction through the AV node and thereby slow ventricular rate. An example of junctional tachycardia is shown in Figure 5-6. The ECG characteristics of this rhythm are shown in Table 5-5.

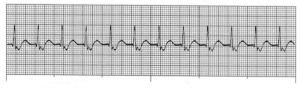

Figure 5-6   Junctional tachycardia at 120 beats/min.

Table 5-5	Characteristics of Junctional Tachycardia
Rhythm	Very regular
Rate	101 to 180 beats/min
P waves	May occur before, during, or after the QRS; if visible, the P wave is inverted in leads II, III, and aVF
PR interval	If a P wave occurs before the QRS, the PR interval will usually be 0.12 sec or less; if no P wave occurs before the QRS, there will be no PR interval
QRS duration	0.11 sec or less unless abnormally conducted

6 Ventricular Rhythms

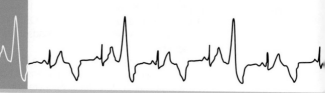

When an ectopic site within a ventricle assumes responsibility for pacing the heart, the electrical impulse bypasses the normal intraventricular conduction pathway. This results in stimulation of the ventricles at slightly different times. As a result, ventricular beats and rhythms usually have QRS complexes that are abnormally shaped and longer than normal (e.g., greater than 0.12 second). If the atria are depolarized after the ventricles, retrograde P waves may be seen.

Because ventricular depolarization is abnormal, ventricular repolarization is also abnormal and results in changes in ST segments and T waves. The T waves are usually in a direction opposite that of the QRS complex; if the major QRS deflection is negative, the ST segment is usually elevated and the T wave positive (i.e., upright). If the major QRS deflection is positive, the ST segment is usually depressed and the T wave is usually negative (i.e., inverted). P waves are usually not seen with ventricular dysrhythmias but if they are visible, they have no consistent relationship to the QRS complex

PREMATURE VENTRICULAR COMPLEXES

A *premature ventricular complex* (PVC) arises from an irritable site within either ventricle. By definition, a PVC is *premature*, occurring earlier than the next expected sinus beat. The shape of the QRS of a PVC depends on the location of the irritable focus within the ventricles (Figure 6-1). The width of the QRS of a PVC is typically 0.12 second or greater because the PVC causes the ventricles to fire prematurely and in an abnormal manner (Figure 6-2). The T wave is usually in a

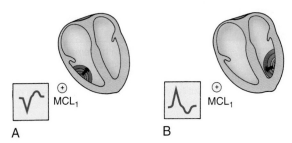

Figure 6-1 **A,** Right ventricular PVC. The spread of depolarization is from right to left, away from the positive electrode in lead V_1 (MCL_1), resulting in a wide, negative QRS complex. **B,** Left ventricular PVC. The spread of depolarization is from left to right, toward the positive electrode in lead V_1 (MCL_1). The QRS complex is wide and upright.

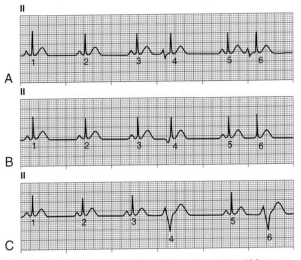

Figure 6-2 Premature beats. **A,** Sinus rhythm with premature atrial complexes (PACs). The fourth and sixth beats are preceded by premature P waves that look different from the normally conducted sinus beats. Note that the QRS complex that follows each of these PACs is narrow and identical in appearance to that of the sinus-conducted beats. **B,** Sinus rhythm with premature junctional complexes (PJCs). The fourth and sixth beats are PJCs. Beat 4 is preceded by an inverted P wave with a short PR interval. There is no identifiable atrial activity associated with beat 6. **C,** Sinus rhythm with PVCs. The fourth and sixth beats are very different in appearance from the normally conducted sinus beats. Beats 4 and 6 are PVCs. They are not preceded by P waves.

Table **6-1**	Characteristics of Premature Ventricular Complexes
Rhythm	Essentially regular with *premature* beats; if the PVC is an interpolated PVC, the rhythm will be regular
Rate	Usually within normal range, but depends on the underlying rhythm
P waves	Usually absent or, with retrograde conduction to the atria, may appear after the QRS (usually upright in the ST segment or T wave)
PR interval	None with the PVC because the ectopic beat originates in the ventricles
QRS duration	Usually 0.12 sec or greater; wide and bizarre; T wave is usually in the opposite direction of the QRS complex

direction that is opposite that of the QRS complex. Most patients experiencing PVCs do not require treatment with antiarrhythmic medications; rather, treatment of PVCs focuses on the search for, and treatment of, potentially reversible causes. For example, provide reassurance to the patient who is complaining of palpitations while searching for possible triggers for his or her PVCs (e.g., excessive caffeine ingestion, nicotine use, emotional stress). The general characteristics of PVCs are shown in Table 6-1.

VENTRICULAR ESCAPE BEATS/RHYTHM

Remember that premature beats are *early* and escape beats are *late*. A ventricular escape beat is a *protective* mechanism. It protects the heart from more extreme slowing or even asystole. Because it is protective, you would not want to administer any medication that would "wipe out" the escape beat. An example of a ventricular escape beat is shown in Figure 6-3. The electrocardiogram (ECG) characteristics of ventricular escape beats are shown in Table 6-2.

An *idioventricular rhythm* (IVR), which is also called a *ventricular escape rhythm*, exists when three or more ventricular

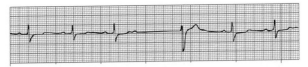

Figure 6-3　Sinus rhythm with a prolonged PR interval, nonconducted PAC, ventricular escape beat, and ST-segment depression.

Table 6-2	Characteristics of Ventricular Escape Beats
Rhythm	Essentially regular with *late* beats; the ventricular escape beat occurs *after* the next expected sinus beat
Rate	Usually within normal range, but depends on the underlying rhythm
P waves	Usually absent or, with retrograde conduction to the atria, may appear after the QRS (usually upright in the ST segment or T wave)
PR interval	None with the ventricular escape beat because the ectopic beat originates in the ventricles
QRS duration	0.12 sec or greater; wide and bizarre; the T wave is frequently in the opposite direction of the QRS complex

escape beats occur in a row at a rate of 20 to 40 beats/min (i.e., the intrinsic firing rate of the Purkinje fibers). The QRS complexes seen in IVR are wide and bizarre because the impulses begin in the ventricles, bypassing the normal conduction pathway. If the patient has a pulse and is symptomatic because of the slow rate, treatment should include application of a pulse oximeter and administration of supplemental oxygen if indicated. Establish intravenous (IV) access, obtain a 12-lead ECG, and administer IV atropine. Reassess the patient's response and continue monitoring the patient. Transcutaneous pacing or a dopamine, epinephrine, or isoproterenol IV infusion may be tried if atropine is ineffective. An example of IVR is shown in Figure 6-4 and the characteristics of this rhythm are described in Table 6-3.

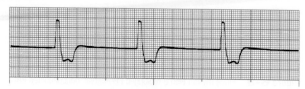

Figure 6-4   Idioventricular rhythm.

Table **6-3**	Characteristics of Idioventricular Rhythm
Rhythm	Ventricular rhythm is essentially regular
Rate	Ventricular rate 20 to 40 beats/min
P waves	Usually absent or, with retrograde conduction to the atria, may appear after the QRS (usually upright in the ST segment or T wave)
PR interval	None
QRS duration	0.12 sec or greater; the T wave is frequently in the opposite direction of the QRS complex

ACCELERATED IDIOVENTRICULAR RHYTHM

An *accelerated idioventricular rhythm* (AIVR) exists when three or more ventricular beats occur in a row at a rate of 41 to 100 beats/min (Figure 6-5). AIVR is usually considered a benign escape rhythm that appears when the sinus rate slows and disappears when the sinus rate speeds up. The ECG characteristics of AIVR are shown in Table 6-4.

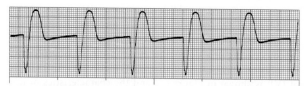

Figure 6-5   Accelerated idioventricular rhythm.

Table **6-4**	Characteristics of Accelerated Idioventricular Rhythm
Rhythm	Ventricular rhythm is essentially regular
Rate	41 to 100 (41 to 120 per some cardiologists) beats/min
P waves	Usually absent or, with retrograde conduction to the atria, may appear after the QRS (usually upright in the ST segment or T wave)
PR interval	None
QRS duration	Greater than 0.12 sec; the T wave is frequently in the opposite direction of the QRS complex

VENTRICULAR TACHYCARDIA

Ventricular tachycardia (VT) exists when three or more sequential PVCs occur at a rate of more than 100 beats/min. VT may occur as a short run that lasts less than 30 seconds and spontaneously ends (i.e., *nonsustained VT*). *Sustained VT* persists for more than 30 seconds and may require therapeutic intervention to terminate the rhythm. VT may occur with or without pulses, and the patient may be stable or unstable with this rhythm.

Monomorphic Ventricular Tachycardia

When the QRS complexes of VT are of the same shape and amplitude, the rhythm is called *monomorphic VT* (Figure 6-6). Treatment is based on the patient's signs and symptoms and the type of VT. If the rhythm is monomorphic VT (and the patient's symptoms are caused by the tachycardia):

- Cardiopulmonary resuscitation (CPR) and defibrillation are used to treat the pulseless patient with VT.
- Stable but symptomatic patients are treated with oxygen (if indicated), IV access, and ventricular antiarrhythmics (e.g., procainamide, amiodarone, sotalol) to suppress the rhythm. Procainamide should be avoided if the patient has a prolonged QT interval or signs of heart failure. Sotalol should also be avoided if the patient has a prolonged QT interval.

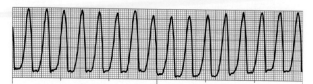

Figure 6-6   Monomorphic ventricular tachycardia.

- Unstable patients (usually a sustained heart rate of 150 beats/min or more) are treated with oxygen, IV access, and sedation (if the patient is awake and time permits) followed by synchronized cardioversion.

In all cases, an aggressive search must be made for the cause of the VT. The ECG characteristics of monomorphic VT are shown in Table 6-5.

Table **6-5**	Characteristics of Monomorphic Ventricular Tachycardia
Rhythm	Ventricular rhythm is essentially regular
Rate	101 to 250 (121 to 250 per some cardiologists) beats/min
P waves	Usually not seen; if present, they have no set relationship with the QRS complexes that appear between them at a rate different from that of the VT
PR interval	None
QRS duration	0.12 sec or greater; often difficult to differentiate between the QRS and T wave

Polymorphic Ventricular Tachycardia

With *polymorphic ventricular tachycardia* (PMVT), the QRS complexes vary in shape and amplitude from beat to beat and appear to twist from upright to negative or negative to upright and back, resembling a spindle. PMVT is a dysrhythmia of intermediate severity between monomorphic VT and ventricular fibrillation (VF) (Figure 6-7). It is best to seek expert

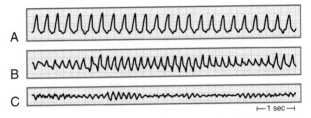

Figure 6-7   Ventricular tachydysrhythmias. **A,** Rhythm strip showing monomorphic VT. **B,** Example of PMVT. **C,** Example of ventricular fibrillation. All tracings are from lead V_1.

consultation when treating the patient with PMVT because of the diverse mechanisms of PMVT, for which there may or may not be clues as to its specific cause at the time of the patient's presentation. In general, if the patient is symptomatic as a result of the tachycardia, treat ischemia (if it is present), correct electrolyte abnormalities, and discontinue any medications that the patient may be taking that prolong the QT interval. If the patient is stable, the use of IV amiodarone (if the QT interval is normal), magnesium, or beta-blockers may be effective, depending on the cause of the PMVT. If the patient is unstable or has no pulse, proceed with defibrillation as for VF. The ECG characteristics of polymorphic VT are shown in Table 6-6.

Table **6-6**	Characteristics of Polymorphic Ventricular Tachycardia
Rhythm	Ventricular rhythm may be regular or irregular
Rate	Ventricular rate 150 to 300 beats/min; typically 200 to 250 beats/min
P waves	None
PR interval	None
QRS duration	0.12 sec or more; there is a gradual alteration in the amplitude and direction of the QRS complexes; a typical cycle consists of 5 to 20 QRS complexes

VENTRICULAR FIBRILLATION

Ventricular fibrillation (VF) is a chaotic rhythm that begins in the ventricles. In VF, there is no organized depolarization of the ventricles. The ventricular muscle quivers, and as a result, there is no effective myocardial contraction and no pulse. The resulting rhythm looks chaotic with deflections that vary in shape and amplitude (see Figure 6-7). No normal-looking waveforms are visible. VF with waves that are 3 or more mm high is called *coarse VF*. VF with low amplitude waves (i.e., less than 3 mm) is called *fine VF*. The priorities of care in cardiac arrest as a result of pulseless VT or VF are high-quality CPR and defibrillation. Medications that may be used in the treatment of pulseless VT/VF include epinephrine, vasopressin, amiodarone, and lidocaine (if amiodarone is unavailable). The ECG characteristics of VF are shown in Table 6-7.

Table **6-7**	Characteristics of Ventricular Fibrillation
Rhythm	Rapid and chaotic with no pattern or regularity
Rate	Cannot be determined because there are no discernible waves or complexes to measure
P waves	Not discernible
PR interval	Not discernible
QRS duration	Not discernible

ASYSTOLE

Asystole, which is also called *ventricular asystole*, is a total absence of ventricular electrical activity (Figure 6-8). There is no ventricular rate or rhythm, no pulse, and no cardiac output. Some atrial electrical activity may be evident. If atrial electrical activity is present, the rhythm is called *"P wave" asystole* or *ventricular standstill*. When asystole is observed on a cardiac monitor, confirm that the patient is unresponsive and has no pulse, and then begin high-quality CPR. Additional care includes establishing vascular access, considering the possible causes of the arrest, administering a vasopressor (e.g., epinephrine, vasopressin), and possibly inserting an advanced airway. The ECG characteristics of asystole are shown in Table 6-8.

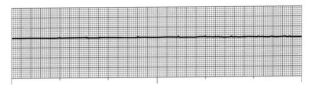

Figure 6-8   Asystole.

Table **6-8**	Characteristics of Asystole
Rhythm	Ventricular not discernible; atrial may be discernible
Rate	Ventricular not discernible but atrial activity may be observed (i.e., "P-wave" asystole)
P waves	Usually not discernible
PR interval	Not measurable
QRS duration	Absent

7

Heart Blocks

ATRIOVENTRICULAR BLOCKS

Depolarization and repolarization are slow in the atrioventricular (AV) node, which makes this area vulnerable to blocks in conduction. When a delay or interruption in impulse conduction from the atria to the ventricles occurs because of a transient or permanent anatomic or functional impairment, the resulting dysrhythmia is called an *AV block*. When analyzing a rhythm strip, disturbances in AV conduction can be detected by assessing PR intervals. The normal PR interval measures 0.12 to 0.20 second.

AV block is classified into (1) first-degree AV block; (2) second-degree AV block (types I and II); and (3) third-degree AV block. With first-degree AV block, impulses from the sinoatrial (SA) node to the ventricles are *delayed*—they are not blocked. With second-degree AV blocks, there is an *intermittent* disturbance in the conduction of impulses between the atria and the ventricles. In third-degree AV block, there is a *complete* block in the conduction of impulses between the atria and the ventricles.

First-degree AV block usually occurs because of a conduction delay within the AV node (Figure 7-1). Second- and third-degree AV blocks can occur at the level of the AV node, the bundle of His, or the bundle branches. AV blocks located at the bundle of His or bundle branches are called *infranodal* or *subnodal* AV blocks.

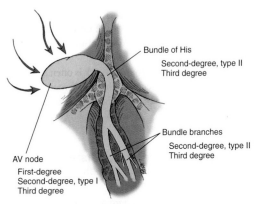

Figure 7-1   Common locations of AV blocks.

First-Degree Atrioventricular Block

With a first-degree AV block, all components of the cardiac cycle are usually within normal limits, with the exception of the PR interval. This is because electrical impulses travel normally from the SA node through the atria, but there is a delay in impulse conduction, usually at the level of the AV node (Figure 7-2). Despite its name, the SA node impulse is not blocked during a first-degree AV block; rather, each sinus impulse is *delayed* for the same period before it is conducted to the ventricles. This delay in AV conduction results in a PR interval that is longer than normal (i.e., more than 0.20 second in duration in adults) and constant before each QRS complex.

First-degree AV block is not a dysrhythmia itself; it is a condition that describes the prolonged (but constant) PR interval

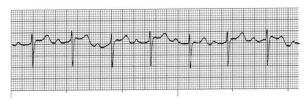

Figure 7-2   Sinus rhythm at 88 beats/min with a first-degree atrioventricular (AV) block and ST-segment elevation.

that is seen on the rhythm strip. Identification of a rhythm strip must include a description of the underlying rhythm, the ventricular rate, and then a description of anything that appears amiss.

The patient with a first-degree AV block is often asymptomatic. First-degree AV block that occurs with acute myocardial infarction (MI) should be monitored closely. The electrocardiogram (ECG) characteristics of first-degree AV block are shown in Table 7-1.

Table **7-1**	Characteristics of First-Degree Atrioventricular Block
Rhythm	Regular
Rate	Usually within normal range, but depends on underlying rhythm
P waves	Normal in size and shape; one positive (upright) P wave before each QRS
PR interval	Prolonged (i.e., more than 0.20 sec) but constant
QRS duration	Usually 0.11 sec or less unless abnormally conducted

Second-Degree Atrioventricular Blocks

The term *second-degree AV block* is used when one or more, but not all, sinus impulses are blocked from reaching the ventricles. Because the SA node generates impulses in a normal manner, each P wave will occur at a regular interval across the rhythm strip (i.e., all P waves will plot through on time), although not every P wave will be followed by a QRS complex. This suggests that the atria are being depolarized normally, but not every impulse is being conducted to the ventricles (i.e., intermittent conduction). As a result, more P waves than QRS complexes are seen on the ECG.

Second-degree AV block is classified as type I or type II, depending on the behavior of the PR intervals associated with the dysrhythmia. The type I or type II designation is used to describe the *ECG pattern* of the PR intervals. The type I or type II designation is used to describe the *ECG pattern* of the PR intervals and should not be used to describe the anatomic site (i.e., location) of the AV block.[1]

Second-Degree Atrioventricular Block Type I

Second-degree AV block type I is also known as *type I block*, *Mobitz I*, or *Wenckebach*. The term *Wenckebach phenomenon* is used to describe a progressive lengthening of conduction time in any cardiac conducting tissue that eventually results in the dropping of a beat or a reversion to the initial conduction time. As each atrial impulse arrives earlier and earlier into the relative refractory period of the impaired AV node, more time is required to conduct the impulse to the ventricles. On the ECG, this is reflected as a progressive increase in the length of the PR intervals (Figure 7-3). When an impulse finally arrives during the AV node's absolute refractory period, it fails to conduct to the ventricles and is seen on the ECG as a P wave that is not followed by a QRS complex. An example of this type of AV block appears in Figure 7-3.

The patient with second-degree AV block type I is usually asymptomatic because the ventricular rate often remains nearly normal and cardiac output is not significantly affected. If the patient is symptomatic and the dysrhythmia is a result of medications (e.g., digoxin, beta-blockers), these substances should be withheld. If the heart rate is slow and serious signs and symptoms occur because of the slow rate, treatment should include applying a pulse oximeter and administering oxygen (if indicated), obtaining the patient's vital signs, and establishing intravenous (IV) access. A 12-lead ECG should be obtained. Atropine, administered intravenously, is the drug of choice. Reassess the patient's response and continue monitoring the patient. ECG characteristics of second-degree AV block type I are shown in Table 7-2.

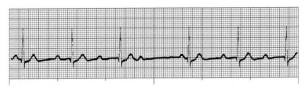

Figure 7-3   Second-degree atrioventricular (AV) block type I at 43 to 60 beats/min.

Table **7-2**	Characteristics of Second-Degree Atrioventricular Block Type I
Rhythm	Ventricular irregular; atrial regular (i.e., Ps plot through on time); grouped beating may be present
Rate	Atrial rate is greater than ventricular rate
P waves	Normal in size and shape; some P waves are not followed by a QRS complex (i.e., more Ps than QRSs)
PR interval	Inconstant; the PR interval after a nonconducted P wave is shorter than the interval preceding the nonconducted beat
QRS duration	Usually 0.11 sec or less; complexes are periodically dropped

Second-Degree Atrioventricular Block Type II

Second-degree AV block type II is also called *type II block* or *Mobitz II* AV block. The conduction delay in second-degree AV block type II occurs below the AV node, within the His-Purkinje system. Most of the time, the block occurs below the bundle of His, which usually produces a wide QRS (i.e., more than 0.11 second in duration).[1] As it is with second-degree AV block type I, there are more P waves than QRS complexes with second-degree AV block type II, and the P waves occur on time. The PR interval with type II block can be normal or prolonged; but it is constant for the conducted beats. Most importantly, the PR intervals before and after a blocked sinus impulse (i.e., P wave) are *constant*.

If the heart rate is slow and serious signs and symptoms occur because of the slow rate, treatment should include applying a pulse oximeter and administering oxygen (if indicated), obtaining the patient's vital signs, and establishing IV access. A 12-lead ECG should be obtained. Although current resuscitation guidelines recommend IV administration of atropine to reduce vagal tone and improve conduction through the AV node, this is effective only if the site of the block is the AV node. If the block is below the AV node, atropine is unlikely to be effective. In this situation, atropine administration will usually not improve the block but rather will increase the rate of discharge of the SA node. This may trigger a situation in which even fewer impulses are conducted through to the ventricles and the ventricular rate is further slowed. Because second-degree AV block type II may abruptly progress to third-degree AV block, the patient should be closely monitored for increasing AV block. When second-degree AV block type II occurs in the setting of an acute anterior MI, temporary or permanent pacing may be necessary. An example of second-degree AV block type II is shown in Figure 7-4. The ECG characteristics of second-degree AV block type II are shown in Table 7-3.

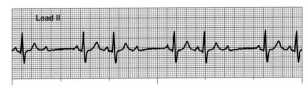

Figure 7-4   Second-degree AV block type II at 48 to 94 beats/min.

Table **7-3**	Characteristics of Second-Degree Atrioventricular Block Type II
Rhythm	Ventricular irregular; atrial regular (i.e., Ps plot through on time)
Rate	Atrial rate is greater than ventricular rate; ventricular rate is often slow
P waves	Normal in size and shape; some P waves are not followed by a QRS complex (i.e., more Ps than QRSs)
PR interval	Within normal limits or prolonged but constant for the conducted beats; the PR intervals before and after a blocked P wave are *constant*
QRS duration	Within normal limits if the block occurs above or within the bundle of His; greater than 0.11 sec if the block occurs below the bundle of His; complexes are periodically absent after P waves

2:1 Atrioventricular Block

With 2:1 AV block, there is one conducted P wave followed by a blocked P wave; thus, two P waves occur for every one QRS complex (i.e., 2:1 conduction). Because there are no two PQRST cycles in a row from which to compare PR intervals, 2:1 AV block cannot be conclusively classified as type I or type II. To determine the type of block with certainty, it is necessary to continue close ECG monitoring of the patient until the conduction ratio of P waves to QRS complexes changes to 3:2, 4:3, and so on, which would enable PR interval comparison.

If the QRS complex measures 0.11 second or less, the block is likely to be located in the AV node and a form of second-degree AV block type I (Figure 7-5). A 2:1 AV block associated with a wide QRS complex (i.e., more than 0.11 second) is usually associated with a delay in conduction below the bundle of His; thus, it is usually a type II block (Figure 7-6). The ECG characteristics of 2:1 AV block are shown in Table 7-4. The causes and emergency management for 2:1 AV block are those of type I or type II block previously described.

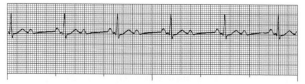

Figure 7-5   Second-degree 2:1 AV block with narrow QRS complexes.

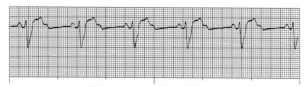

Figure 7-6   Second-degree 2:1 AV block with wide QRS complexes.

Table 7-4	Characteristics of Second-Degree 2:1 Atrioventricular Block
Rhythm	Ventricular regular; atrial regular (Ps plot through on time)
Rate	Atrial rate is twice the ventricular rate
P waves	Normal in size and shape; every other P wave is not followed by a QRS complex (i.e., more Ps than QRSs)
PR interval	Constant
QRS duration	May be narrow or wide; complexes are absent after every other P wave

Advanced Second-Degree Atrioventricular Block

The terms *advanced* or *high-grade* second-degree AV block may be used to describe three or more consecutive P waves that are not conducted. For example, with 3:1 AV block, every third P wave is conducted (i.e., followed by a QRS complex); with 4:1 AV block, every fourth P wave is conducted (Figure 7-7).

As is the case with 2:1 AV block, advanced second-degree AV block cannot be conclusively classified as type I or type II because there are no two PQRST cycles in a row from which to compare PR intervals. Monitoring of the patient's ECG for changes in P wave to QRS conduction ratios to enable PR interval comparison is essential. Because of the frequency with which impulses from the SA node to the Purkinje fibers are blocked, the presence of advanced AV block is a cause for concern and the development of third-degree AV block should be anticipated.

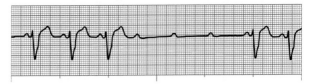

Figure 7-7   An example of advanced second-degree AV block.

Third-Degree Atrioventricular Block

Second-degree AV blocks are types of *incomplete* blocks because at least some of the impulses from the SA node are conducted to the ventricles. With third-degree AV block, there is a *complete* block in conduction of impulses between the atria and the ventricles. The site of block in a third-degree AV block may be the AV node or, more commonly, the bundle of His or the bundle branches (Figure 7-8). A secondary pacemaker (either junctional or ventricular) stimulates the ventricles; therefore, the QRS may be narrow or wide, depending on the location of the escape pacemaker and the condition of the intraventricular conduction system. The ECG characteristics of third-degree AV block are shown in Table 7-5.

The patient's signs and symptoms will depend on the origin of the escape pacemaker (i.e., junctional versus ventricular) and the patient's response to a slower ventricular rate. If the patient

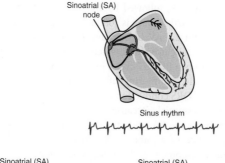

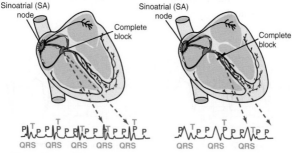

Figure 7-8   Third-degree AV block. AV, atrioventricular; SA, sinoatrial.

Table **7-5**	Characteristics of Third-Degree Atrioventricular Block
Rhythm	Ventricular regular; atrial regular (Ps plot through); no relationship between the atrial and ventricular rhythms (i.e., atrioventricular (AV) dissociation is present)
Rate	The ventricular rate is determined by the origin of the escape rhythm; the atrial rate is greater than (and independent of) the ventricular rate; ventricular rate is determined by the origin of the escape rhythm
P waves	Normal in size and shape; some P waves are not followed by a QRS complex (i.e., more Ps than QRSs)
PR interval	None: the atria and the ventricles beat independently of each other, thus there is no true PR interval
QRS duration	Narrow or wide, depending on the location of the escape pacemaker and the condition of the intraventricular conduction system

is symptomatic because of the slow rate, treatment should include applying a pulse oximeter and administering oxygen (if indicated), obtaining the patient's vital signs, establishing IV access, and obtaining a 12-lead ECG. IV administration of atropine may be tried. If the disruption in AV nodal conduction is caused by increased parasympathetic tone, the administration of atropine may be effective in reversing excess vagal tone and improving AV node conduction. Other interventions that may be used in the treatment of third-degree AV block include epinephrine, dopamine, or isoproterenol IV infusions, or transcutaneous pacing. Frequent patient reassessment is essential. Most patients with third-degree AV block have an indication for permanent pacemaker placement.

INTRAVENTRICULAR CONDUCTION DELAYS[2]

During normal ventricular depolarization, the left side of the interventricular septum is stimulated first. The electrical impulse (i.e., wave of depolarization) then traverses the septum to stimulate the right side. The left and right ventricles are then depolarized at the same time (Figure 7-9). *A bundle branch block* (BBB) is a disruption in impulse conduction from the bundle of His through either the right or left bundle branch to the Purkinje fibers. A BBB may be intermittent or permanent, complete or incomplete.

If a delay or block occurs in one of the bundle branches, the ventricles will not be depolarized at the same time. The impulse first travels down the unblocked branch and stimulates that ventricle. Because of the block, the impulse must then travel from cell to cell through the myocardium (rather than through the normal conduction pathway) to stimulate the other ventricle. This means of conduction is slower than normal, and the QRS complex appears widened on the ECG. The ventricle with the blocked bundle branch is the last to be depolarized.

Essentially two conditions must exist to suspect BBB. First, the QRS complex must have an abnormal duration (i.e., 0.12 second or more in width if a complete BBB), and second, the QRS complex must arise as the result of supraventricular activity (this excludes ventricular beats). If these two conditions are met, delayed ventricular conduction is assumed to be present, and BBB is the most common cause of this abnormal conduction.

With BBB, the last ventricle to be depolarized is, of course, the ventricle with the blocked bundle branch. Therefore, if it is

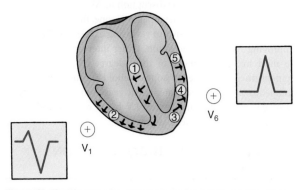

Figure 7-9 Sequence of normal ventricular depolarization and resulting QRS complex, as seen in leads V_1 and V_6.

possible to determine the ventricle that was depolarized last, it becomes possible to determine the bundle branch that was blocked. For example, if the right ventricle was depolarized last, it is because the impulse travelled down the left bundle branch, depolarized the left ventricle first, then marched through and depolarized the right ventricle. It stands to reason that if one ventricle is depolarized late, its depolarization makes up the later portion of the QRS complex.

The final portion of the QRS complex is referred to as the *terminal force*. Examination of the terminal force of the QRS complex reveals the ventricle that was depolarized last, and, therefore, the bundle that was blocked. To identify the terminal force, first locate the J point. From the J point, move backward into the QRS and determine if the last electrical activity produced an upward or downward deflection. An example of the terminal force in both right bundle branch block (RBBB) and left bundle branch block (LBBB) is illustrated in Figure 7-10. If the right bundle branch is blocked, then the right ventricle will be depolarized last and the current will be moving from the left ventricle to the right. This will create a positive deflection of the terminal force of the QRS complex in V_1. If the left bundle branch is blocked, the left ventricle will be depolarized last, and the current will flow from right to left. This will produce a negative deflection of the terminal force of the QRS complex seen in V_1. Therefore, to differentiate RBBB from LBBB, look at V_1 and determine whether the terminal force of the QRS complex is a positive or negative deflection. If it is directed upward, an RBBB is present (i.e., the current is moving toward the right ventricle and toward V_1). A LBBB is present when the terminal force of the QRS complex is directed downward (i.e., the current is moving away from V_1 and toward the left ventricle). This rule is especially helpful when rSR′ and QS variants are present. A simple way to remember this rule has been suggested by Mike Taigman and Syd Canan, and is demonstrated in Figure 7-11. They recognized the similarity between this rule and the turn indicator on a car. When a right turn is made, the turn indicator is lifted up. Likewise, when a RBBB is present, the terminal force of the QRS complex points up. Conversely, left turns and LBBB are directed downward. Unfortunately not every BBB presents with a clear pattern as

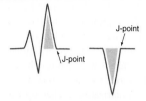

J-point

J-point

Figure 7-10 Determining the direction of the terminal force. In lead V$_1$, move from the J point into the QRS complex and determine whether the terminal portion (last 0.04 second) of the QRS complex is a positive (upright) or negative (downward) deflection.

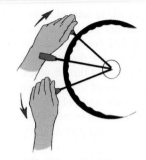

Figure 7-11 Differentiating between right and left bundle branch blocks. The "turn signal" theory is that right is up and left is down.

previously described, which makes the differentiation between right and left BBB less clear.

The presence of a BBB in an asymptomatic patient requires no specific treatment. Right BBB generally requires no specific treatment; however, when RBBB occurs in the setting of an acute MI, close ECG monitoring for the development of symptomatic AV conduction system disturbances is essential. Because of its association with organic heart disease, the patient with LBBB should be evaluated for cardiomyopathies, coronary disease, hypertension, valvular heart disease, and other conditions associated with LBBB. Insertion of a permanent pacemaker is generally required for patients with LBBB who develop second-degree AV block type II or third-degree AV block.

Exceptions[2]

Two notable exceptions must be mentioned to complete the discussion of BBB. The first involves the criteria used to recognize BBB, and the second relates to differentiating LBBB from RBBB.

The criteria used to recognize BBB are valid but lack some sensitivity and specificity. The sensitivity can be limited by junctional rhythms because there may be no discernible P waves when the AV junction is the pacemaker site. The AV junction is a supraventricular pacemaker, but this presents as an exception to the two-part rule of BBB recognition. Specificity is limited by Wolff-Parkinson-White (WPW) syndrome and other conditions that produce wide QRS complexes resulting from atrial activity. If the characteristic delta wave and shortened PR interval are recognized, WPW syndrome should be suspected.

As for differentiating LBBB from RBBB, a third category exists: *nonspecific intraventricular conduction delay* (NSIVCD). These blocks do not display the typical V_1 morphologies generally produced by BBB. Their origin may not be the result of a complete BBB but are often the result of several factors, of which incomplete BBB may be one. Atypical patterns of BBB can be attributed to NSIVCD.

Pacemaker Rhythms

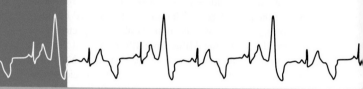

INTRODUCTION

A cardiac pacemaker is a battery-powered device that delivers an electrical current to the heart to stimulate depolarization. A pacemaker system consists of a *pulse generator* (i.e., the power source) and pacing leads. The pulse generator houses a battery and electronic circuitry. The circuitry works like a computer, converting energy from the battery into electrical pulses. A lithium battery is usually the power source for implanted pacemakers and implantable cardioverter-defibrillators (ICDs), whereas a 9-volt alkaline battery is usually used to power a temporary external pulse generator. A *pacing lead* is an insulated wire that is used to carry an electrical impulse from the pulse generator to the patient's heart. It also carries information about the heart's electrical activity back to the pacemaker. The pacemaker responds to the information received either by sending a pacing impulse to the heart (i.e., *triggering*) or by not sending a pacing impulse to the heart (i.e., *inhibition*).

PERMANENT PACEMAKERS AND IMPLANTABLE CARDIOVERTER-DEFIBRILLATORS

A permanent pacemaker is used to treat disorders of the sinoatrial (SA) node (e.g., bradycardias), disorders of the atrioventricular (AV) conduction pathways (e.g., second-degree AV block type II, third-degree AV block), or both, that produce signs and symptoms as a result of inadequate cardiac output.

The pacemaker's pulse generator is usually implanted under local anesthesia into the subcutaneous tissue of the anterior chest just below the right or left clavicle.

An ICD is a programmable device that can deliver a range of therapies (also called *tiered-therapy*) including defibrillation, antitachycardia pacing (i.e., *overdrive pacing*), synchronized cardioversion, and bradycardia pacing, depending on the dysrhythmia detected and how the device is programmed. A physician determines the appropriate therapies for each patient.

TEMPORARY PACEMAKERS

The pulse generator of a temporary pacemaker is located externally. Temporary pacing can be accomplished through transvenous, epicardial, or transcutaneous means.

Transvenous pacemakers stimulate the endocardium of the right atrium or ventricle (or both) by means of an electrode introduced into a central vein, such as the subclavian, femoral, brachial, internal jugular, or external jugular vein. Epicardial pacing is the placement of pacing leads directly onto or through the epicardium. Epicardial leads may be used when a patient is undergoing cardiac surgery and the outer surface of the heart is easy to reach.

Transcutaneous pacing (TCP) delivers pacing impulses to the heart using large electrodes that are placed on the patient's chest. TCP is also called *temporary external pacing* or *noninvasive pacing*. TCP is indicated for significant bradycardias that are unresponsive to atropine therapy or when atropine is not immediately available or indicated. It may also be used as a bridge until transvenous pacing can be accomplished or the cause of the bradycardia is reversed (e.g., drug overdose, hyperkalemia). *Standby pacing* refers to the application of the pacing pads to the patient's chest in anticipation of possible use, but pacing is not yet needed. For example, standby pacing is often warranted when second-degree AV block type II or third-degree AV block are present in the setting of acute myocardial infarction (MI). The range of output current of a transcutaneous pacemaker varies depending on the manufacturer. You must be familiar with your equipment before you need to use it.

PACING LEAD SYSTEMS

Pacemaker lead systems may consist of single, double, or multiple leads. The exposed portion of the pacing lead is called an *electrode*, which is placed in direct contact with the heart. Pacing, which is also called *pacemaker firing*, occurs when the pacemaker's pulse generator delivers energy (milliamperes [mA]) through the pacing electrode to the myocardium. Evidence of pacing can be seen as a vertical line or spike on the electrocardiogram (ECG).

Capture is the successful conduction of an artificial pacemaker's impulse through the myocardium, resulting in depolarization. Capture is obtained after the pacemaker electrode is properly positioned in the heart; with one-to-one capture, each pacing stimulus results in depolarization of the appropriate chamber. On the ECG, evidence of *electrical capture* can be seen as a pacemaker spike followed by an atrial or a ventricular complex, depending on the cardiac chamber that is being paced. *Mechanical capture* is assessed by palpating the patient's pulse or by observing right atrial pressure, left atrial pressure, or pulmonary artery or arterial pressure waveforms.

A unipolar electrode has one pacing electrode that is located at its distal tip. The negative electrode is in contact with the cardiac tissue, and the pulse generator (located outside the heart) functions as the positive electrode. The pacemaker spike produced by a unipolar lead system is often large because of the distance between the positive and negative electrode. Unipolar leads are less commonly used than bipolar lead systems because of the potential for pacing the chest wall muscles and the susceptibility of the unipolar leads to electromagnetic interference.

A bipolar lead system contains a positive and negative electrode at the distal tip of the pacing lead wire (Figure 8-1). Most temporary transvenous pacemakers use a bipolar lead system. A permanent pacemaker may have either a bipolar or a unipolar lead system. The pacemaker spike produced by a bipolar lead system is smaller than that of a unipolar system because of the shorter distance between the positive and negative electrodes.

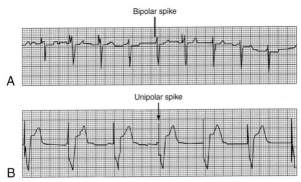

Figure 8-1 Bipolar and unipolar pacing. **A,** Pacemaker spike produced by a bipolar lead system. **B,** Pacemaker spike produced by a unipolar lead system.

Single-Chamber Pacemakers

A pacemaker that paces a single heart chamber, either the atrium or ventricle, has one lead placed in the heart. Atrial pacing is achieved by placing the pacing electrode in the right atrium. Stimulation of the atria produces a pacemaker spike on the ECG, followed by a P wave (Figure 8-2). Atrial pacing may be used when the SA node is diseased or damaged, but conduction through the AV junction and ventricles is normal. This type of pacemaker is ineffective if an AV block develops because it cannot pace the ventricles.

Ventricular pacing is accomplished by placing the pacing electrode in the right ventricle. Stimulation of the ventricles produces a pacemaker spike on the ECG followed by a wide QRS, resembling a ventricular ectopic beat (Figure 8-3). The

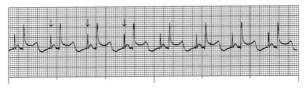

Figure 8-2 Electrocardiogram of a single-chamber pacemaker with atrial pacing spikes (arrows).

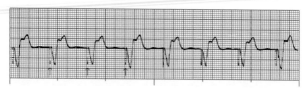

Figure 8-3 Electrocardiogram of a single-chamber pacemaker with ventricular pacing spikes (arrows).

QRS complex is wide because a paced impulse does not follow the normal conduction pathway in the heart. A single-chamber ventricular pacemaker can pace the ventricles but it cannot coordinate pacing with the patient's intrinsic atrial rate. This results in asynchronous contraction of the atrium and ventricle (i.e., AV asynchrony). Because of this loss of AV synchrony, a ventricular demand pacemaker is rarely used in a patient with an intact SA node. Conversely, a ventricular demand pacemaker may be used for the patient with chronic atrial fibrillation.

Dual-Chamber Pacemakers

A dual-chamber pacemaker uses two leads: one lead is placed in the right atrium and the other in the right ventricle. Dual-chamber pacing is also called *physiologic pacing*. A dual-chamber pacemaker stimulates the right atrium and right ventricle sequentially (stimulating first the atrium, then the ventricle), mimicking normal cardiac physiology and thus preserving the atrial contribution to ventricular filling (i.e., atrial kick) (Figure 8-4).

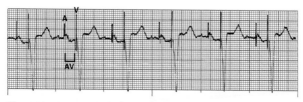

Figure 8-4 Electrocardiogram of a dual-chamber pacemaker with atrial pacing spikes (A), ventricular pacing spikes (V). AV, AV interval.

Biventricular Pacemakers

A *biventricular pacemaker* has three leads; one lead for each ventricle and one lead for the right atrium. This device uses cardiac resynchronization therapy to restore normal simultaneous ventricular contraction for patients with heart failure, thereby improving cardiac output and exercise tolerance.

Fixed-Rate Pacemakers

A *fixed-rate pacemaker*, which is also known as an *asynchronous* pacemaker, continuously discharges at a preset rate (usually 70 to 80 impulses/min) regardless of the patient's heart rate or metabolic demands. An advantage of the fixed-rate pacemaker is its simple circuitry, reducing the risk of pacemaker failure; however, this type of pacemaker does not sense the patient's own cardiac rhythm. This may result in competition between the patient's cardiac rhythm and that of the pacemaker. Ventricular tachycardia or ventricular fibrillation may be induced if the pacemaker were to fire during the T wave (i.e., the vulnerable period) of a preceding patient beat. Fixed-rate pacemakers are not often used today.

Demand Pacemakers

A *demand pacemaker*, which is also known as a *synchronous* or *noncompetitive* pacemaker, discharges only when the patient's heart rate drops below the pacemaker's base rate. For example, if the demand pacemaker was preset at a base rate of 70 impulses/min, it would sense the patient's heart rate and allow electrical impulses to flow from the pacemaker through the pacing lead to stimulate the heart only when the rate fell below 70 beats/min. Demand pacemakers can be programmable or nonprogrammable. The voltage level and impulse rate are preset at the time of manufacture in nonprogrammable pacemakers.

PACEMAKER CODES

Pacemaker codes are used to assist in identifying a pacemaker's preprogrammed pacing, sensing, and response functions (Table 8-1). The *first letter* of the code identifies the heart chamber (or chambers) paced (stimulated). A pacemaker used to pace only a single chamber is represented by either A (atrial) or

Table **8-1**	Revised NASPE/BPEG* Generic Code for Antibradycardia Pacing				
Position	**I**	**II**	**III**	**IV**	**V**
Category	Chamber(s) Paced	Chamber(s) Sensed	Response to Sensing	Rate Modulation	Multisite Pacing
	O = None	O = None	O = None	O = None	O = None
	A = Atrium	A = Atrium	T = Triggered	R = Rate Modulation	A = Atrium
	V = Ventricle	V = Ventricle	I = Inhibited		V = Ventricle
	D = Dual (A + V)	D = Dual (A + V)	D = Dual (T + I)		D = Dual (A + V)
Manufacturer's Designation Only	S = Single (A or V)	S = Single (A or V)			

From Bernstein A, Daubert J, Fletcher R, Hayes D, et al: The revised NASPE/BPEG generic code for antibradycardia, adaptive-rate, and multisite pacing. North American Society of Pacing and Electrophysiology/British Pacing and Electrophysiology Group, Pacing Clin Electrophysiol 2002;25(2):260-264.

*NASPE/BPEG, North American Society of Pacing and Electrophysiology/British Pacing and Electrophysiology Group.

V (ventricular). A pacemaker capable of pacing in both chambers is represented by D (dual). The *second letter* identifies the chamber of the heart where patient-initiated (i.e., intrinsic) electrical activity is sensed by the pacemaker. The *third letter* indicates how the pacemaker will respond when it senses patient-initiated electrical activity. The *fourth letter* identifies the availability of rate modulation (i.e., the pacemaker's ability to adapt its rate to meet the body's needs caused by increased physical activity and then increase or decrease the pacing rate accordingly). A pacemaker's rate modulation capability may also be referred to as *rate responsiveness* or *rate adaptation*. The *fifth letter* denotes multisite pacing.

A defibrillator code was developed in 1993 and it is used to describe the capabilities and operation of ICDs (Table 8-2).

Table 8-2   NASPE/BPEG* Defibrillator Codes

Position I	Position II	Position III	Position IV
Shock Chamber	Antitachycardia Pacing Chamber	Tachycardia Detection	Antibradycardia Pacing Chamber
O = None	O = None	E = Electrogram	O = None
A = Atrium	A = Atrium	H = Hemodynamic	A = Atrium
V = Ventricle	V = Ventricle		V = Ventricle
D = Dual (A + V)	D = Dual (A + V)		D = Dual (A + V)

From Bernstein AD, Camm AJ, Fisher JD, Fletcher RD, et al: North American Society of Pacing and Electrophysiology policy statement: the NASPE/BPEG defibrillator code, Pacing Clin Electrophysiol 1993;16:1776-1780.

*NASPE/BPEG, North American Society of Pacing and Electrophysiology/British Pacing and Electrophysiology Group.

Introduction to the 12-Lead ECG

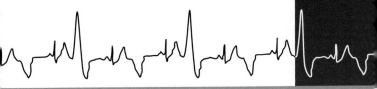

INTRODUCTION

A standard 12-lead electrocardiogram (ECG) provides views of the heart in both the frontal and horizontal planes and views the surfaces of the left ventricle from 12 different angles. Multiple views of the heart can provide useful information including the following:

- Identification of ST-segment and T-wave changes associated with myocardial ischemia, injury, and infarction
- Identification of ECG changes associated with certain medications and electrolyte imbalances
- Recognition of bundle branch blocks

Indications for using a 12-lead ECG include the following:

- Assisting in dysrhythmia interpretation
- Chest pain or discomfort
- Electrical injuries
- Known or suspected electrolyte imbalances
- Known or suspected medication overdoses
- Right or left ventricular failure
- Status before and after electrical therapy (e.g., defibrillation, cardioversion, pacing)
- Stroke
- Syncope or near syncope
- Unstable patient, unknown etiology

VECTORS

Leads have a negative (−) and positive (+) electrode pole that senses the magnitude and direction of the electrical force caused by the spread of waves of depolarization and repolarization throughout the myocardium.

A *vector* (arrow) is a symbol representing this force. A vector points in the direction of depolarization. Leads that face the tip or point of a vector record a positive deflection on ECG paper. A *mean vector* identifies the average of depolarization waves in one portion of the heart. The *mean P vector* represents the average magnitude and direction of both right and left atrial depolarization. The *mean QRS vector* represents the average magnitude and direction of both right and left ventricular depolarization. The average direction of a mean vector is called the *mean axis* and is only identified in the frontal plane. An imaginary line joining the positive and negative electrodes of a lead is called the *axis* of the lead. *Electrical axis* refers to determining the direction, or angle in degrees, in which the main vector of depolarization is pointed.

Axis

During normal ventricular depolarization, the left side of the interventricular septum is stimulated first. The electrical impulse then traverses the septum to stimulate the right side. The left and right ventricles are then depolarized simultaneously. Because the left ventricle is considerably larger than the right, right ventricular depolarization forces are overshadowed on the ECG. As a result, the mean QRS vector points down (i.e., inferior) and to the left.

Axis determination can provide clues in the differential diagnosis of wide QRS tachycardia and localization of accessory pathways. In adults, the normal QRS axis is considered to be between −30 and +90 degrees in the frontal plane. Current flow to the right of normal is called *right axis deviation* (between +90 and ±180 degrees). Current flow in the direction opposite of normal is called *indeterminate,* "no man's land," *northwest,* or *extreme right axis deviation* (−90 and ±180 degrees). Current flow to the left of normal is called *left axis deviation* (between −30 and −90 degrees).

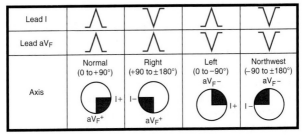

Lead I				
Lead aVF				
Axis	Normal (0 to +90°)	Right (+90 to ±180°)	Left (0 to −90°) aVF−	Northwest (−90 to ±180°) aVF−

Figure 9-1 Determination of QRS axis quadrant by noting predominant QRS polarity in leads I and aVF. Normal axis: If the QRS is primarily positive in both I and aVF, the axis falls within the normal quadrant from 0 to 90 degrees. Right axis deviation: If the QRS complex is primarily negative in I and positive in aVF, right axis deviation is present. Left axis deviation: If the QRS complex is predominantly positive in I and negative in aVF, left axis deviation is present. Indeterminate axis: If the QRS is primarily negative in both I and aVF, a markedly abnormal "indeterminate" or "northwest" axis is present.

Shortcuts exist to determine axis deviation. Leads I and aVF divide the heart into four quadrants. These two leads can be used to quickly estimate electrical axis. In leads I and aVF, the QRS complex is normally positive. If the QRS complex in either or both of these leads is negative, axis deviation is present (Figure 9-1).

ACUTE CORONARY SYNDROMES

You will recall from Chapter 1 that acute coronary syndromes (ACSs) are conditions caused by a similar sequence of pathologic events and involve a temporary or permanent blockage of a coronary artery. ACSs include unstable angina, non–ST-(segment) elevation myocardial infarction (NSTEMI), and ST-(segment) elevation myocardial infarction (STEMI). Sudden cardiac death can occur with any of these conditions.

ST-Elevation Myocardial Infarction

Recognition of infarction on the ECG relies on the detection of morphologic changes (i.e., changes in shape) of the QRS complex, the T wave, and the ST segment. These changes occur in relation to certain events during the infarction.

Non–ST-Elevation Myocardial Infarction

As its name implies, patients experiencing a NSTEMI do not show signs of myocardial injury (ST-segment elevation) on their ECG. The diagnosis of NSTEMI is made based on the patient's signs and symptoms, history, and cardiac biomarker test results that confirm the presence of an infarction. If serum biomarkers are not present in the patient's circulation based on two or more samples collected at least 6 hours apart, the diagnosis is unstable angina. If elevated biomarker levels are present, the diagnosis is NSTEMI.

Localization of Infarctions

ECG changes of myocardial ischemia, injury, or infarction are considered significant if they are viewed in two or more anatomically contiguous leads. If these ECG findings are seen in leads that look directly at the affected area, they are called *indicative changes*. If findings are seen in leads opposite the affected area, they are called *reciprocal changes* (Figure 9-2).

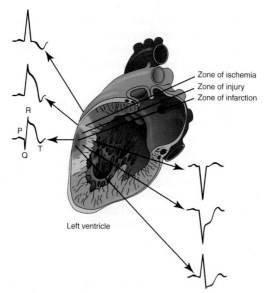

Figure 9-2 Zones of ischemia, injury, and infarction showing indicative ECG changes and reciprocal changes corresponding to each zone.

Leads II, III, and aVF view the inferior wall of the left ventricle. Because these leads "see" the same part of the heart, they are considered contiguous leads. Leads I, aVL, V_5, and V_6 are contiguous because they all look at adjoining tissue in the lateral wall of the left ventricle. Leads V_1 and V_2 are contiguous because both leads look at the septum. Leads V_3 and V_4 are contiguous because both leads look at the anterior wall of the left ventricle. If right chest leads such as V_4R, V_5R, and V_6R are used, they are contiguous because they view the right ventricle. Leads V_7, V_8, and V_9 are contiguous because they look at the posterior surface of the heart.

PREDICTING THE SITE OF CORONARY ARTERY OCCLUSION[2]

In the standard 12-lead ECG, leads II, III, and aVF "look" at tissue supplied by the right coronary artery. Eight leads "look" at tissue supplied by the left coronary artery: leads I, aVL, V_1, V_2, V_3, V_4, V_5, and V_6. When evaluating the extent of infarction produced by a left coronary artery occlusion, decide how many of these leads are showing indicative changes. The more of these eight leads that show indicative changes, the larger the infarction is presumed to be.

The left ventricle has been divided into regions where a myocardial infarction (MI) may occur: septal, anterior, lateral, inferior, and inferobasal (i.e., posterior) (Figure 9-3). If an ECG shows changes in leads II, III, and aVF, the inferior wall is affected. Because the inferior wall of the left ventricle is supplied by the right coronary artery in most people, it is reasonable to suppose that these ECG changes are caused by partial or complete blockage of the right coronary artery. When indicative changes are seen in the leads viewing the septal, anterior, and/or lateral walls of the left ventricle (i.e., V_1-V_6, I, and aVL), it is reasonable to suspect that these ECG changes are caused by partial or complete blockage of the left coronary artery.

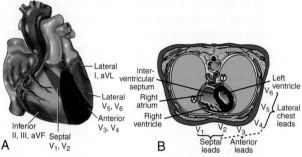

Figure 9-3 **A,** The surfaces of the heart. The inferobasal (posterior) surface is not shown. **B,** The areas of the heart as seen by the chest leads. Leads V_1, V_2, and V_3 are contiguous. Leads V_3, V_4, and V_5 are contiguous as well as V_4, V_5, and V_6. Note that neither the right ventricular wall (X) nor the inferobasal surface of the left ventricle (Y) is well visualized by any of the usual six chest leads.

ANALYZING THE 12-LEAD ELECTROCARDIOGRAM

The following five-step approach is recommended when reviewing a 12-lead ECG[2]:

1. *Identify the rate and underlying rhythm.* Determining rate and rhythm is the first priority when interpreting the ECG. Remember, the treatment of life-threatening dysrhythmias initially takes precedence over the acquisition and interpretation of the 12-lead ECG. If baseline wander or artifact is present to any significant degree, note it. If the presence of either of these conditions interferes with the assessment of any lead, use a modifier such as "possible" or "apparent" in your interpretation.

2. *Analyze waveforms.* Examine each lead, selecting one good representative waveform or complex in each lead. Examine each lead for the presence of a wide Q wave. If a Q wave is present, express the duration in milliseconds. Next, look for the presence of ST-segment displacement (i.e., elevation or depression). Elevation of the ST segment is the most reliable marker during the first hours of

infarction and may be recognizable before significant tissue loss has occurred. Therefore, each lead, with the exception of aVR, should be examined for the presence of indicative changes with special emphasis on ST-segment elevation and pathologic Q waves. Evidence must be found in at least two anatomically contiguous leads. If ST-segment elevation is present, express it in millimeters. Examine the T waves for any changes in orientation, shape, and size. Note the presence of tall, peaked T waves or T-wave inversion.

3. *Examine for evidence of infarction.* Is a STEMI suspected? What is the location? If ST-segment displacement is present, assess the areas of ischemia or injury by assessing lead groupings. If acute MI is suspected, mentally picture the cardiac anatomy to localize the infarction and predict which coronary artery is occluded. The relative extent of the infarction can be gauged by the number of leads showing ST-segment elevation. Remember that in suspected right coronary artery occlusions, right-sided chest leads should be obtained to help gauge the extent of the infarct and identify possible right ventricular infarction. Please note that more advanced 12-lead interpretation generally includes a careful analysis of R-wave progression and axis deviation, among other factors. In this text, our focus is on the identification of ECG findings suggestive of acute MI.

4. *Ascertain if STEMI imposters are present that may account for ECG changes.* When changes indicative of an acute infarction are noted on the ECG, ascertain if other conditions are present that might also account for the changes. In cases where these conditions are present, do not rule out infarction, but recognize that these ECG changes may be a result of infarction or one of the infarct impostors (e.g., left ventricular hypertrophy, left bundle branch block, ventricular rhythm, ventricular paced rhythm). Remember, infarction can still occur in the presence of each of these conditions. Therefore, when you are screening potential infarct patients, recognition of indicative changes in the presence of one of the infarct impostors warrants an immediate physician over-read (i.e., careful physician review and interpretation of the 12-lead ECG).

5. *Make a STEMI decision.* On the basis of your ECG findings, decide if clear evidence is present that a STEMI exists: (1) A STEMI is definitely not present, (2) a suspected STEMI is present, and (3) possible STEMI (i.e., a STEMI imposter is present, making interpretation difficult).

Illustration Credits

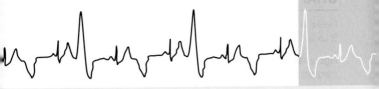

CHAPTER 1

Figures 1-1, 1-2, 1-6   Drake R: *Gray's anatomy for students,* ed 2, New York, 2010, Churchill Livingstone.

Figures 1-3 to 1-5   Thibodeau GA, Patton, KT: *Anatomy and physiology,* ed 7, St Louis, 2010, Mosby.

Figure 1-7   Herlihy B, Maebius NK: *The human body in health and illness,* ed 3, St Louis, 2007, Mosby.

CHAPTER 2

Figure 2-1   Koeppen BM: *Berne and Levy physiology,* ed 6, updated edition, St Louis, 2010, Mosby.

Figure 2-2   Costanzo LS: *Physiology,* ed 4, Philadelphia, 2010, Saunders.

Figures 2-3, 2-6 to 2-8, 2-11   Copstead-Kirkhorn LEC: *Pathophysiology,* ed 4, Philadelphia, 2009, Saunders.

Figures 2-4, 2-15   Crawford MV, Spence MI: *Common sense approach to coronary care,* rev ed 6, St Louis, 1994, Mosby.

Figure 2-5, 2-12   Boron WF: *Medical physiology,* ed 2, Philadelphia, 2012, Saunders.

Figure 2-9   Drew BJ, Ide B: Right ventricular infarction, *Prog Cardiovasc Nurs* 1995;10:46.

Figure 2-10   AACN: *AACN procedure manual for critical care,* ed 6, Philadelphia, 2011, Saunders.

Figures 2-13, 2-14 Urden LD: *Critical care nursing: diagnosis and management,* ed 6, St Louis, 2012, Mosby.

CHAPTER 4

Figure 4-2 Kinney MR: *Andreoli's comprehensive cardiac care,* ed 8, St Louis, 1996, Mosby.

Figure 4-4 Paul S, Hebra JD: *The nurse's guide to cardiac rhythm interpretation: implications for patient care,* Philadelphia, 1998, Saunders.

Figure 4-5 Braunwald E, Zipes DP: *Heart disease: a textbook of cardio-vascular medicine,* ed 6, Philadelphia, 2001, Saunders.

Figures 4-6, 4-8 Goldberger AL: *Clinical electrocardiography: a simplified approach,* ed 7, St Louis, 2006, Mosby.

Figure 4-10 Surawicz B, Knilans T: *Chou's electrocardiography in clinical practice: adult and pediatric,* ed 6, Philadelphia, 2008, Saunders.

CHAPTER 5

Figure 5-1 Grauer K: *A practical guide to ECG interpretation,* ed 2, St Louis, 1998, Mosby.

CHAPTER 6

Figure 6-1 Urden LD: *Critical care nursing: diagnosis and management,* ed 6, St Louis, 2012, Mosby.

Figure 6-2 Grauer K: *A practical guide to ECG interpretation,* ed 2. St Louis, 1998, Mosby.

Figure 6-3 Surawicz B, Knilans T: *Chou's electrocardiography in clinical practice: adult and pediatric,* ed 6, Philadelphia, 2008, Saunders.

Figure 6-7 Goldman, L, Ausiello DA, Arend W, et al: *Cecil medicine,* ed 23, Philadelphia, 2007, Saunders.

CHAPTER 7

Figures 7-4, 7-7 Aehlert B: *ECGs made easy study cards,* St Louis, 2004, Mosby.

Figure 7-7 Urden LD: *Critical care nursing: diagnosis and management,* ed 6, St Louis, 2012, Mosby.

References

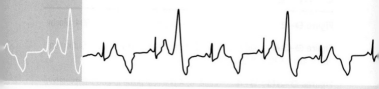

1. Barold SS, Hayes DL: Second-degree atrioventricular block: a reappraisal, *Mayo Clin Proc* 2001;76(1):44-57.
2. Phalen T, Aehlert B: *The 12-lead ECG in acute coronary syndromes,* ed 3, St. Louis, 2012, Elsevier, pp 75-161.

Index

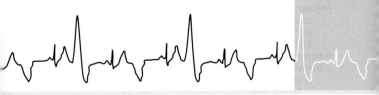